SECOND EDITION

# PROJECT PLANNING AND MANAGEMENT

## A Guide for Nurses and Interprofessional Teams

**James Harris,**
**PhD, APRN-BC, MBA, CNL, FAAN**
Professor, University of South Alabama
Birmingham, Alabama

**Linda Roussel,**
**DSN, RN, NEA-BC, CNL**
DNP Program Coordinator and Professor
University of South Alabama
Birmingham, Alabama

**Catherine Dearman, PhD, RN**
Professor/Associate Dean,
Research and Evaluation
College of Nursing
University of South Alabama
Mobile, Alabama

**Patricia L. Thomas,**
**PhD, RN, NEA BC, CNL**
Director, Nursing Practice & Research
Trinity Health
Detroit, Michigan

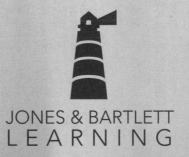

JONES & BARTLETT
LEARNING

*World Headquarters*
Jones & Bartlett Learning
5 Wall Street
Burlington, MA 01803
978-443-5000
info@jblearning.com
www.jblearning.com

Jones & Bartlett Learning books and products are available through most bookstores and online booksellers. To contact Jones & Bartlett Learning directly, call 800-832-0034, fax 978-443-8000, or visit our website, www.jblearning.com.

**Production Credits**

VP, Executive Publisher: David D. Cella
Executive Editor: Amanda Martin
Associate Acquisitions Editor: Rebecca Myrick
Editorial Assistant: Danielle Bessette
Associate Production Editor: Kristen Rogers
Director of Marketing: Alisha Weisman
Senior Marketing Manager: Jennifer Scherzay
Production Services Manager: Colleen Lamy
VP, Manufacturing and Inventory Control:
Therese Connell
Composition: S4Carlisle Publishing Services
Cover Design: Michael O'Donnell
Media Development Assistant: Shannon Sheehan
Rights and Media Research Assistant: Wes DeShano
Cover Image: © Jim Lopes/ShutterStock, Inc.
Printing and Binding: Edwards Brothers Malloy
Cover Printing: Edwards Brothers Malloy

**Library of Congress Cataloging-in-Publication Data**

Project planning and management (Harris)
  Project planning and management : a guide for nurses and interprofessional teams / [edited by] James Harris, Linda Roussel, Patricia (Tricia) Thomas, Catherine Dearman. —Second edition.
    p. ; cm.
  Preceded by: Project planning and management : a guide for CNLs, DNPs, and nurse executives / edited by James L. Harris ... [et al.]. c2011.
  Includes bibliographical references and index.
  ISBN 978-1-284-08983-7 (pbk.)
  I. Harris, James L. (James Leonard), 1956- , editor. II. Roussel, Linda, editor. III. Thomas, Patricia L., 1961- , editor. IV. Dearman, Catherine, editor. V. Title.
  [DNLM: 1.  Nursing—organization & administration. 2.  Nursing Research—methods. 3.  Interprofessional Relations. 4.  Planning Techniques. 5.  Program Development—methods. WY 105]
  RT89
  610.73068—dc23
                        2015019681
6048
Printed in the United States of America
19  18  17  16  15    10  9  8  7  6  5  4  3  2  1

# TABLE OF CONTENTS

# PREFACE

The primary function of a textbook is to be a reference source for students, educators, practitioners, and administrators. As healthcare organizations are challenged to maintain a competitive edge, meaningful projects that add value, contribute evidence, and are sustainable will be required. Our dedication and commitment as educators, administrators, clinicians, and researchers led us to update the content from the first edition of this text, *Project Planning and Management: A Guide for CNLs, DNP, and Nurse Executives*, as projects are a constant activity in all organizations. As care environments continue to require the most up-to-date information and innovative practices, interprofessional project teams and learning collaboratives have formed. The collective talents and insight of these teams are needed to meet the challenges inherent in providing quality, safe, and efficient care. As interprofessional project teams work together, new behaviors develop and an understanding of various disciplines emerges as projects progress.

We contend that the content in the *Second Edition* is not all-inclusive, but rather provides guideposts for interprofessional teams as they design, update, and evaluate innovative projects that will transcend all care settings. This edition's content lays the foundation for successful project planning and management, interprofessional team management techniques, implementation science, team synergy, and use of clinical needs assessments to shape projects. The value of information and measurement is also highlighted throughout this text. Based on comments from students, faculty, and institutional review boards, we also added material (in two separate chapters) on the need to differentiate research and quality improvement projects as well as the criteria for approving each for data collection and future dissemination.

We hope that the information provided in this *Second Edition* will encourage interprofessional teams to engage in meaningful projects and to become advocates for interprofessional team engagement, learning collaboratives, and care environments that continuously strive to meet the myriad demands and challenges in today's dynamic healthcare systems. A committed team can and will set the stage necessary for advancing knowledge in a culture of lifelong learning and sharing.

James L. Harris
Linda Roussel
Catherine Dearman
Patricia L. Thomas

# ACKNOWLEDGMENTS

My colleagues and I acknowledge each of the contributors to this text and the mentors who have guided our careers. In an era of constant changes in health care, the call for transformative leaders to support interprofessional teams as they engage in value-added projects is a timely one. Effective projects create new venues for patient-centered care and opportunities for team synergy where knowledge is generated that will guide novel evidence-based practice.

To our families and colleagues who supported this endeavor, we thank you for the encouragement. To our colleagues at Jones & Bartlett Learning, your unwavering direction and support is greatly appreciated.

James L. Harris
Linda Roussel
Catherine Dearman
Patricia L. Thomas

# CONTRIBUTORS

**Murielle S. Beene, DNP, RN-BC, MBA, MPH, MS, PPH, PMP**
Chief Nursing Informatics Officer
Department of Veterans Affairs
Washington, DC

**Michael Bleich, PhD, RN, FAAN**
President and Dean
Goldfarb School of Nursing at Barnes-
   Jewish College
St. Louis, Missouri

**Catherine Dearman, PhD, RN**
Professor of Nursing
Associate Dean of Research and
   Development
University of South Alabama
Mobile, Alabama

**Frank Weston Garrison, IV, MSN, RN, MBA, NE-BC**
Chief Nursing Officer
CHI St. Luke's Health System
Sugar Land, Texas

**Todd Harlan, DNP, RN**
Associate Professor of Nursing
Chair, Community Mental Health
   Nursing
University of South Alabama
Mobile, Alabama

**James L. Harris, PhD, APRN-BC, MBA, CNL, FAAN**
Professor of Nursing
University of South Alabama
Mobile, Alabama

**Carolynn Thomas Jones,
DNP, MSPH**
Lead Instructor, Master of Applied
  Clinical and Preclinical Research
Assistant Professor of Nursing, College
  of Nursing
The Ohio State University
Columbus, Ohio

**Theodora Ledford, MSN, RN, CNL**
Former CNL Student, University
of South Alabama
Asheville, North Carolina

**Summer Li, MSHA, PMP**
Program Leader
Trinity Health
Livonia, Michigan

**Jacqueline M. Lollar, DNP, RN**
Assistant Professor of Nursing
Chair, Maternal Child Nursing
University of South Alabama
Mobile, Alabama

**K. Michele Lyons, MN**
Southeastern Louisiana University
Hammond, Louisiana

**Andrew Missel, MPH**
Program Manager, Clinical Quality
  and Operations
CHE Trinity Health
Livonia, Michigan

**Margaret Mitchell, MN, FNP**
Graduate Student, University of South
  Alabama
Mobile, Alabama

**Terri Poe, DNP, RN**
Chief Nursing Officer
University of Alabama Hospital
Birmingham, Alabama

**Shea Polanchich, PhD, RN**
Assistant Professor of Nursing
University of Alabama at Birmingham
Birmingham, Alabama

**Linda Roussel, PhD, RN, NEA-BC**
Professor of Nursing and Coordinator,
  Doctor of Nursing Program
University of Alabama at Birmingham
Birmingham, Alabama

**Jennifer Styron, PhD**
Assistant Professor
University of South Alabama
Mobile, Alabama

**Ronald A. Styron, Jr., PhD**
Quality Enhancement Director
  and Professor
University of South Alabama
Mobile, Alabama

**Heather Surcouf, DNP Student**
Southeastern Louisiana University
Hammond, Louisiana

**Patricia L. Thomas, PhD, RN,
NEA-BC, CNL**
Vice President Clinical Quality
  and Transformation
Chief Nursing Officer
Trinity Home Health Services
Livonia, Michigan

**Kathryn M. Ward-Presson, DNP, RN,
NEA-BC**
Executive Healthcare Consulting, LLC
Jonas Scholar in Veterans Healthcare Alumni
Raleigh, North Carolina

**Sheila Whitworth, DNP, RN**
Assistant Professor
University of South Alabama
Mobile, Alabama

## CHAPTER ONE

# Key Foundations of Successful Project Planning and Management

*James L. Harris*

## *Chapter Objectives*

1. Differentiate between a project, a plan, and their management.
2. Prioritize needs to support a project plan and program sustainability.
3. Combine the components of project planning to design a value-based program.
4. Identify requisite skills and tools for the development, initiation, evaluation, and dissemination of quality improvement projects and their continuous management.
5. Generate processes necessary to manage individuals and system-wide projects and teams in virtual environments.

## *Key Terms*

| | | |
|---|---|---|
| Continuous quality improvement | Project management | Value |
| Management | Stakeholders | Virtual environment |
| Project plan | Sustainability | |
| | Teams | |

## *Roles*

| | | |
|---|---|---|
| Communicator | Educator | Manager |
| Designer | Leader | |

## *Professional Values*

| | |
|---|---|
| Integrity | Patient-centeredness |

## *Core Competencies*

| | | |
|---|---|---|
| Analysis | Critical thinking | Integration |
| Appreciative inquiry | Emotional intelligence | Risk anticipation and mitigation |
| Assessment | Evidence-based practice | |
| Communication | Leadership | Systems thinking |

# Introduction

Regardless of the industry, transformation is central to the future success of a global economy. What was once merely pondered by many in the healthcare arena has evolved into sustainable project plans and value-based programs that are driven by the basic instinct of survival. New vistas of appreciative inquiry await a mindful revolution of individuals and global leaders dedicated to seamless integration and coordination of projects that will ultimately benefit the health and economic well-being of society (Robert Wood Johnson, 2014).

As individuals consider the daunting task of improving health and well-being at the micro level of a global society, they must recognize that having a project idea and actually implementing it are two different things. Understanding the scope of a project, the stakeholder involvement, team dynamics, and the actual requirements can lead many to become daunted and enter a state of paralysis. In the healthcare industry, the path to an innovative project that will add **value** from the micro level and potentially globally centers around six elements as identified by the World Health Organization (WHO, 2008):

1. Addressing the service to be delivered
2. Financing
3. Governance
4. Workforce
5. Information systems
6. Supply management

Successful planning and implementation of any project are supported by the notion that effective system strengthening requires systems thinking and attention to how the parts work together to create a seamless whole (Crisp, 2010). As knowledge is gained from project outcomes, knowledge transfer becomes an imperative. Evidence is spread and systems of care are strengthened and sustained. This is relevant in the current environment, where the focus of work is on obtaining the right outcomes, as opposed to past decades, where performing the right processes was emphasized (Porter-O'Grady & Malloch, 2015).

This chapter focuses on differences in a project, the project plan, the project's **management**, and strategies used to prioritize project needs. Linking value to the project design, requisite skills, and tools necessary for a successful and sustainable project are then described. As work environments continue to become more virtual, managing project **teams** remotely also becomes a concern; such virtual management is discussed in this chapter as well.

## Projects, Project Plans, and Project Management Defined

The genesis of any project is planning, but ongoing management of the project is essential as well. All projects have a beginning, an end, and a duration, which collectively constitute the project's life cycle. Project outcomes may be, for example, adopted in the form of evidence-based guidelines or seen as opportunities to conduct additional inquiry and validation studies prior to including them in practice. It is critical, however, not to immediately adopt findings from a small project, as they may not be generalizable to a broader context. According to Peters (1999), approximately 50% of the work completed in organizations may be considered as projects. Many staff working on projects as de facto members or managers may not possess the critical path and earned value analysis skills key to orchestrating and managing a project from inception to completion (Lewis, 2011).

What is a project? According to the Project Management Institute (2013), a project is a temporary endeavor focused on producing a unique operational entity (e.g., a product, a service, or a result differing from that obtained in prior projects). Juran (1992) describes a project as a problem scheduled for solution. While the word "problem" may elicit a negative emotion, it does not necessarily imply negativity. Outcomes can create a positive problem, such as a new product or clinical procedure directed at reducing urinary tract infections among elderly individuals or addressing other clinical phenomena. In any event, the project should be based on the notion of accomplishing a goal for systems, **stakeholders**, and/or customers.

When does the project begin? A series of activities and actions precedes the initiation of a project. One fundamental consideration is readying the project environment by identifying and validating the need for the project, developing the plan, and obtaining system buy-in and/or approval from stakeholders.

A **project plan** encompasses several components that collectively culminate in a realistic and well-planned sequence of actions and processes. The project plan goes beyond a general project scope and includes the details necessary to make a meaningful and value-based addition to a work unit or an entire system. According to Tuthill (2014), the project plan includes a budget, a work and activity breakdown and schedule, an overall project schedule, and any supporting documents. Haughey (2009) identified other, but related parts of the project plan, including project goals, deliverables, schedule, and supporting documents (human resources, communications, and risk management plans). Additionally, other project plan considerations were outlined by Billows (2014), whose project plan template provides for scope definition, major deliverables, risk identification, team resource requirements, and decomposing individual tasks. A variety of project-planning programs are available commercially and often used by larger, more complex projects within systems.

Thinking and rethinking what one needs or desires in relation to the project plan are key aspects of planning captured by Merrifield (2009). This author identified three important "rethinking questions" for any student or project planning team:

1.    Does the project exactly correlate with any of the organization's key business goals?
2.    Does the project have a strong connection to the organization's brand or corporate identity?
3.    Does the effort required for the project result in increased organizational performance and change the value of the project to achieve organizational effectiveness?

What is **project management**? The *Project Management Book of Knowledge (PMBOK) Guide* defines project management as "application of knowledge, skills, tools, and techniques to project activities to meet project requirements. Project management is accomplished through the application and integration of the project management processes of initiating, planning, executing, monitoring and controlling, and closing" (Project Management Institute, 2013, p. 6). Of interest, the *PMBOK Guide* has as its primary objective the explanation of how each of the processes may be accomplished in practice.

While consistent management of activities is essential for project completion, project management extends beyond managing and scheduling activities. Project management entails a combination of tools, people, and systems (Lewis, 2011). Tools may include computers, software packages, and daily planners. People include organizations and project teams who engage in processes geared toward goal accomplishment within systems. Management of people may present as a challenge in this endeavor, and leaders and communicators must use multiple skills to coach and mentor individuals toward achieving the common goal. The manager's emotional intelligence may be tested along the way, as will be discussed further in this chapter.

Regardless of the depth or breadth of the project, plan, and management, the various stages of the project life cycle must not be neglected. Tuthill (2014) identified this cycle as having four phases:

1. Initiating the project (including identifying customer-driven factors and obtaining leadership approval and support)
2. Planning (including human and physical resources)
3. Executive (monitors, control, and cycle of effort(s)
4. Project closure (training, operations, and support)

Project planning across the life cycle should also take into account the project's feasibility, value, key drivers for success, skills and tools needed, and processes whereby project teams may be managed in **virtual environments**.

## Prioritizing Needs That Support Project Plans and Programs

The challenges facing the healthcare industry today are complicated by rising expenditures, quality and safety concerns, changes in service needs and expectations, new technologies, provider shortages, and care reform legislation, to name a few of the myriad influences in this environment. In such a complex and rapidly changing landscape, identifying what needs to be done and determining how to quickly accomplish a task is essential if projects are supported, sustained, and manageable, and if they are to truly impact organizations and programs. To ensure effectiveness of a project, one must start by prioritizing the primary need and any evidentiary basis that underpins a need for change and rapid response. Otherwise, the feasibility of any project will be jeopardized from its inception.

Which steps should a student or project team take to prioritize needs? An assessment of the environment is an initial step, which is then followed by development of a strategy. Strategy planning must include consideration of any unintended consequences of the project. This requires the identification of "what if" scenarios and solutions with projected and/or desired measurable outcomes.

## Assessing the Environment

New circumstances require a "new state" that is not known and must emerge from development of a vision, innovation, and learning. Such an effort requires a fundamental shift in mindset, organizing principles, behavior, culture, and infrastructure. A critical mass within the organization or work unit must operate from a new mindset and behavior if change is to be achieved.

A prudent individual who is beginning to develop a project plan must also be aware of the constancy of change. Change is not necessarily a linear or sequential process, but rather may appear at any point during an environmental assessment. Scholars have gleaned much from studies of complex adaptive systems in relation to change. Specifically, change cannot be specified and managed in detail. Small changes in critical elements or leverage points, however, have the potential to engender large changes. Leadership, values, and culture are important for achieving any change, whether that change is implemented by a student engaging in a capstone project or through a system-wide initiative (Plsek & Greenhalgh, 2001). Change can have a profound impact on developing the best strategy necessary to initiate and complete a project. Being attuned to emerging conditions, forces, and trends may provide an individual with insight into the convergence of subtleties that create and affect work environments and the readiness for change (Porter-O'Grady & Malloch, 2015).

When assessing the environment, two fundamental activities should occur sequentially: an assessment of strengths, weaknesses, opportunities, and threats (SWOT analysis) and a gap analysis. Input from both the SWOT analysis and the gap analysis are used in all systems. Output from one type of analysis can be

**Table 1-1**    SWOT and Gap Analysis: Uses in Health Care

| SWOT Analysis | Gap Analysis |
|---|---|
| Hospital comparison data | Patient discharge by 11 A.M. |
| Eliminate hospital-acquired pressure ulcers (Zero HAP Program) | Reduce emergency department wait times by:<br>• 15% in Quarter 1<br>• 75% in Quarters 2–4<br>• 90% for fiscal year |
| Build comprehensive cardiac care center | Streamline waits for elective cardiac studies |

used as input for the other, and vice versa. In completing the SWOT analysis, all levels (micro, meso, and macro) must be examined, as information from each area can provide valuable insights when delimiting the scope of the project and strategies to control positive and negative factors affecting success.

Closely linked to the SWOT analysis is the gap analysis, in which individuals seek to establish the root problem and collect evidence that supports the need for engaging in the project. A gap analysis compares actual performance with potential performance, such as that demonstrated via performance measures. This type of analysis may also be referred to as a needs assessment. During the gap analysis, the current state of the system, factors needed to reach a target or benchmark, and a plan to fill the gap may be identified. This type of assessment is very beneficial in all systems, but especially in today's healthcare arena, where the impetus is on identifying areas with performance deficits that impact resource allocation, planning, productivity, and quality indicators.

Both SWOT analysis and gap analysis are useful to a system, and their findings can be drilled down to identify a common denominator. Indeed, both types of analyses can be used in different contexts with different meanings. **Table 1-1** describes the different uses of each from a healthcare perspective.

## *Strategy Development*

Upon completion and analysis of the SWOT and gap analysis, the strategy is selected and developed to address the priority need(s). As noted by Lewis (2011), strategy is the overall approach to a problem. Strategy is very important because it is often possible to generate multiple alternative solutions to a problem. It is not uncommon for students to take away differing ideas from assessment data and then find themselves conflicted about which problem to tackle first. Should the problem selected be of personal interest, rather than based on system needs? This type of question is why strategy is so important.

In the situation where several problems are identified (based on personal preference and system need), one technique is to rank order them by engaging a team for their prioritization. Engaging others in the process engenders buy-in and ownership of a successful project. Consideration should be given to the environmental assessment, various variables, and data points available in this process.

The selected strategy should also address various levels of need—micro, meso, and macro system needs—depending on the scope of the project. Many healthcare systems today maintain a list of quality improvement projects at a variety of levels needing intervention, as suggested by root-cause analysis findings, internal focused reviews, and/or external reviews. Regardless of whether a "wish list" of projects is provided, any student engaged in a capstone project should complete the environmental assessment and strategy development steps. This creates opportunities for gleaning new information and learning more about the process—knowledge that will prove useful when the student is engaged in or leading projects.

As previously stated, anticipating unintended consequences and managing them to achieve measurable and desired outcomes are steps that cannot be ignored. Unanticipated and unintended consequences are present in all environments. Many such consequences can be traced to prior decisions and attempts to solve problems without projecting those actions' long-range consequences or providing for risk mitigation. It is human nature to want to do the right thing. Without careful analysis of issues and engagement of stakeholders, however, situations may occur that have deleterious effects. Risk anticipation and mitigation are therefore needed, as is identification of ways to avoid and overcome problems, while preserving the intent and integrity of the project.

Good communication at all levels is a cornerstone of successful projects. Consensus on a final project that is clearly presented and mutually agreed upon is needed before the project starts. Many individuals and project teams present a succinct project plan or business case in a concise format. Gaining the support of team members and all stakeholders early on in the process becomes essential to the ongoing sustainability of the project, as ultimately programs depend on both individual and collective input. Milestones must be detailed and met, though these points may be communicated in different ways.

## Value-Based Project Attributes for Project Sustainment and Management

The healthcare system in the United States remains the most costly in all developed countries, with healthcare expenditures expected to increase from 17% to 20% of the gross domestic product by 2020 (Centers for Medicare and Medicaid Services, 2010). Regardless of the country, however, all health systems are challenged to create greater value from the resources dedicated to health care (Institute for Healthcare Improvement [IHI], 2014). Porter-O' Grady and Malloch (2015) contend that clinical work processes today must derive value from a purpose directed toward a desired outcome and emphasize work that achieves real value, rather than focusing on the work itself. Achieving high value for patients must be the primary goal for any project. If value improves, all stakeholders can benefit, and the economic sustainability of programs and the healthcare system will, in turn, increase (Porter, 2010).

Since value is expressed relative to costs, efficiency and accountability should be shared among all individuals involved. This reinforces the need to involve others in any project, concentrating on integrated activities where all stakeholders are accountable for value-based outcomes (Porter, 2010). Projects planned with the IHI Triple Aim (IHI, 2014) in mind can optimize health system performance and engage other stakeholders. But why consider the Triple Aim when planning projects? The dimensions of the Triple Aim—namely, improving the patient's experience of care, improving population health, and reducing the per-capita cost of care—are foundational to harnessing a broad range of community determinants of health and services, where others are engaged and a seamless journey of care follows. As projects are planned and all components are considered, adopting a strategy that will achieve the Triple Aim can be realized as solutions to problems are identified further upstream, beyond the inpatient setting. Fundamentally, the value proposition of the project, thought of mathematically as "Value = Quality/Cost," extends beyond a unit or acute care setting to community-based care (Lighter, 2011). Ideally, the burden of illness is decreased through coordinated care and the per-capita costs are stabilized or reduced.

Well-designed projects with measurable outcomes solidify evidence-based practice and support further inquiry. One means to project value that is commonly used by organizations, accrediting and certification agencies, and students is the six industry services characteristics highlighted by the Institute of Medicine (IOM):

1. Safe
2. Effective
3. Patient-centered
4. Timely
5. Efficient
6. Equitable (IOM, 2001; Steinwachs & Hughes, 2008)

Regardless of how small or large the project is, all well-developed and well-executed projects are driven by key markers of value and success. These key markers include innovation, inclusiveness, an evidence-based foundation, and transparency. New innovative practices and technology are spurred daily by individual and group brainstorming, which often serves as the originating point for value-driven projects that sustain effective programs. Including others in any project idea and design can only enhance outcomes and provide more stakeholders who want to be a part of the planned change. Otherwise, enthusiasm for projects may deteriorate rapidly, and what was initially recognized as a need or gap may become lost in the shuffle. All projects and their design should have solid supporting evidence and be guided by sound methods with rigor, keeping in mind the strategy and ultimate deliverables. Transparency cannot be emphasized enough with any project plan, design, implementation, and dissemination of outcomes. From a project's inception through its end point, remaining open and communicating progress engenders the spirit of ownership necessary for the final outcomes of the value-based project to be readily adopted by programs.

## Skills and Tools as Contributors to Meaningful Projects

In the fast-paced, ever-changing healthcare landscape, a plethora of skills and tools are needed throughout the life cycle of a project, but especially quality improvement ones. Envisioning a future state where the path forward can readily be recognized and followed by others is a deliberate action that leads to meaningful projects and supports their sustained management. The ability to manage the delicate dance of leading, engaging, and inspiring others toward greatness is one of the many skills needed by a project designer and manager. Investment in skill development and core competencies for project planning and management is central to shaping business outcomes in all industries, but especially health care. Applying human factors engineering in health care allows one to gain the knowledge needed to examine human behavior and interaction with others or with their surroundings, and apply information for greater efficacy (Gosbee & Anderson, 2003). Human factors engineering can further assist both the novice and expert project planner and manager in gaining insight into processes quickly and being able to initiate actions for course correction, as applicable.

The skills and tools needed for success with a project include an array of critical techniques and approaches. While there is no singular set of skills and tools that guarantees success, some options are mutually beneficial to individuals and organizations. The process for instilling these skills and tools into practice requires first understanding each and then linking it to goals and measurable, sustainable outcomes. Examples of skills and tools will be provided in this text, keeping in mind none is necessarily better than—or a replacement for—another.

Throughout an improvement project, keeping activities focused on the customers is important, especially when the organization depends on those customers for revenue and the majority of its market share. When customers are satisfied, loyalty is preserved and repeat business occurs. For example, if a manager requests the development of a quality improvement project that will increase customer satisfaction, it is important to first understand customer needs and expectations (understanding gleaned through the assessment process) and then to communicate those needs and expectations throughout the organization, while measuring value and reporting results.

Every project requires a designated leader to establish the direction of and ultimate goal for the project. While there may be informal leaders, the project leader should possess the skills needed to create and maintain the environment where others engage in meeting the project's goal. Creating opportunities to inspire others and involve them in both the current project and future projects is a mark of transformational leaders, who continually encourage and recognize others' contributions.

Being an effective communicator will engage others and provide the leverage necessary to initiate and complete projects in an expeditious fashion. However, this outcome will not occur without the ability, awareness, and sensitivity to address cultural differences in today's highly diverse workforce. All individuals process information differently due to their different cultural backgrounds and beliefs. Being aware and sensitive can facilitate progress on projects (Seibert, Trejo, & Zimmerman, 2002).

Planning and organizational skills, such that one can assimilate information from various assessment processes and break down information into discrete parts, can set the stage for effective ongoing management of the project. Individual creativity may flourish when these skills are applied to organize outcomes for dissemination.

## Managing Projects and Teams in a Virtual Environment

One of the great rewards of technology is the opportunity to have global project team members contribute remotely. Project managers can leverage the strengths and talents of multiple individuals that match the project plan, strategy, and desired outcomes. As Porter-O'Grady and Malloch (2015) explain, teams are small systems and often mirror the complexity in other levels of the larger system. The effectiveness and performance of a project team, whether virtual or not, are contingent upon a combination of attributes and skill sets. These personal assets include individual competence, interpersonal skills, flexibility, accommodation, creativity, strong work ethic, and an outcomes focus, to name a few. If the team has no identified purpose or end point, there is no meaning to the work to be accomplished. Projects may fail or yield limited outcomes that are not sustainable, and future virtual teams may be considered suspect.

As the moral compass for the virtual team, the leader should bring gentle diplomacy to bear in the discourse with staff, managers, stakeholders, and/or distractors. In particular, it is the virtual team leader's responsibility to defend the project and virtual team by shielding the overarching goal from distractors (Sturmberg & Martin, 2012). Adaptability becomes pivotal to success and is often more important than anticipation in such an environment.

Managing a virtual team can be rewarding as well as challenging. Virtual Hires (2014) identified nine guidelines that apply when selecting and managing individuals and teams in virtual environments:

1. Perform a project evaluation. Project leaders must be knowledgeable about goals, tactics, and deliverables if they are to communicate effectively with prospective team members.

2. Determine the skill sets needed by team members. Match the skills of team members to the delegated tasks and mutually reach consensus on assignments. Leveraging individual strengths promotes measurable outcomes.

3. Identify and anticipate obstacles. Knowing what has been attempted previously to resolve a problem or opportunity can only benefit the present outcomes. Conversely, disregarding this information can mean a loss for the plan, as the strategy may actually require only a minor redesign or assignment of a team member with matching skills and competencies.

4. Constantly engage members and encourage bidirectional communication. Contact with virtual team members often is employed to verify needs for supervision and encouragement. Likewise, the team member can communicate successes and challenges encountered that require intervention.

5. Establish a timeline and milestones. Identify expectations and the schedule needed to move the project toward completion. Monitor progress at designated intervals. Share accomplishments with all virtual members and stakeholders.

6.  Ensure individual team member accountability. Recognizing the importance of each individual member's investment in achieving the critical priorities of a specific project and his or her buy-in to the larger institutional performance is a critical success factor.
7.  Be cognizant of cultural differences. Being aware and sensitive to the diversity of virtual team members is important to avoid conflicts and delays in completing assigned tasks.
8.  Manage conflict and difficult team members. Avoiding a conflict will only perpetuate the issue and result in inefficiency of the individual and team function. Although crucial conversations may be difficult on a personal level, they are valuable for resolution of identified issues that may create project paralysis.
9.  Provide education and training. Just-in-time or accelerated learning techniques may be required to assure all team members are on the same page with respect to the project goal and strategies. Using practical application examples and techniques matched with evidence, flexibility, and innovative teaching strategies can strengthen project outcomes and create synergy among virtual team members.

Effective governance and ownership of any project is critical to success. A poorly articulated and organized management structure, overlapping roles and decision-making authority, and mismatched roles and team members can prevent a project from achieving any momentum or producing valuable outcomes. The designated leader is the guardian of a finite project, who is charged with creating the structure and practices needed to guide the plan forward and strategically align it with the enterprise's overall direction.

Virtual teams hold much promise in the healthcare arena, where changing reimbursement models and movement toward greater industry transparency have placed substantial pressure on organizations to deliver stronger performance and improved value. In the long term, this trend is expected to continue. In turn, current improvements and projects focused on cost and quality performance will impel healthcare organizations toward higher standards requiring visionary leaders and dedicated project teams positioned to meet the challenges facing the healthcare industry.

## Summary

- Planning successful projects requires a series of deliberate and purposeful activities that result in an attainable goal.
- Projects may be limited to the micro system or may extend to the meso and macro system level(s) within an organization or industry.
- Projects are finite in scope, whereas program management extends across a system or industry.
- Leadership is central to successful projects and their sustainability.
- Projects that include the Triple Aim goals will benefit both systems and stakeholders.
- Envisioning a futuristic state opens up avenues for changes in behavior and value-based project outcomes.
- Technology affords opportunities for global project team membership where talents are leveraged toward an achievable goal.

## Reflection Questions

1. Reflect on your current work environment and identify how leaders within the organization impact project successes, sustained practice change, and spread of evidence.
2. Identify and discuss a technological advance that may assist you as a capstone project is developed and implemented. Which technology might help you evaluate the project's impact within a healthcare system?
3. Which attributes contribute to a virtual project team's success? How can you ensure positive changes and outcomes as the project leader?

## References

Billows, D. (2014). Project plan template: How to create a project plan. http://4pm.com/project-plan-template/

Centers for Medicare and Medicaid Services. (2010). Affordable Care Act update: Improving Medicare cost savings. http://www.cms.gov/apps/docs/aca-update

Crisp, N. (2010). *Turning the world upside down: The search for global health in the 21st century.* London, UK: RSM Press.

Gosbee, J., & Anderson, T. (2003). Human factors engineering design demonstrations can enlighten your RCA team. *Quality Safe Healthcare, 12,* 119–121.

Haughey, D. (2014). Project planning a step by step guide. http://www.projectsmart.com/articles/project-planning-a-step-by-step-guide.php

Institute for Healthcare Improvement (IHI). (2014). The IHI Triple Aim. http://www.ihi.org.Engage/Initiatives/TripleAIM/Pages/default.aspx

Institute of Medicine (IOM). (2001). *Crossing the quality chasm: A new health system for the 21st century.* Washington, DC: National Academy Press.

Juran, J. M. (1992). *Juran on quality by design.* New York, NY: Simon and Schuster.

Lewis, J. P. (2011). *Project planning, scheduling and control: The ultimate hands-on guide to bringing projects in on time and on budget* (5th ed.). New York, NY: McGraw-Hill.

Lighter, D. M. (2011). *Advanced performance improvement in health care.* Sudbury, MA: Jones and Bartlett.

Merrifield, R. (2009). *Re-think.* Upper Saddle River, NJ: Pearson.

Peters, T. (1999). *The wow project.* San Francisco, CA: Fast Company. http://www.fastcompany.com/36831/wow-project

Plsek, P. E., & Greenhalgh, T. (2001). The challenge of complexity in healthcare. *British Medical Journal, 323,* 625–628.

Porter, M. E. (2010). What is value in health care? *New England Journal of Medicine, 363,* 2477–2481.

Porter-O'Grady, T., & Malloch, K. (2015). *Quantum leadership: Building better partnerships for sustainable health.* Burlington, MA: Jones & Bartlett Learning.

Project Management Institute. (2013). *A guide to project management body of knowledge (PM-BOK guide)* (5th ed.). Newtown Square, PA: Author.

Robert Wood Johnson Foundation. (2014). Time to act: Investing in the health of our children and communities. Recommendations from the Robert Wood Foundation Commission to Build a Healthier America executive summary. http://www.rwjf.org

Seibert, P. S., Trejo, L. S., & Zimmerman, C. G. (2002). A checklist to facilitate cultural awareness and sensitivity. *Journal of Medical Ethics, 28,* 143–146.

Steinwachs, D. M., & Hughes, R. G. (2008). Health services research: Scope and significance. In R. G. Hughes (Ed.), *Patient safety and quality: An evidence-based handbook for nurses* (Vol. 1), 163–177. Rockville, MD: Agency for Healthcare Research and Quality.

Sturmberg, J. P., & Martin, C. M. (2012). Leadership and transitions: Maintaining the science in complexity and complex systems. *Journal of Evaluation and Clinical Practice, 18,* 186–189.

Tuthill, J. M. (2014). *Practical project management for informatics! How to manage a project without losing your mind.* Presentation at API Annual Conference, Chicago, IL.

Virtual Hires. (2014). 15 tips for effectively mapping your virtual employee. http://www.virtual-hires.com/resources.cgi?file=15-tips-to-effectively-managing-your-virtual-employee

World Health Organization (WHO). (2008). *Closing the gap in a generation: Health equity through action on the social determinants of health. Commission on Social Determinants of Health.* New York, NY: Author.

# Case Exemplar

## ■ CASE STUDY 1

### Guidepost for Students Selecting a Meaningful Capstone Project Topic

*Jacqueline Lollar*

As a former labor and delivery nurse in a teaching hospital and a current nurse educator, Sandy had always wanted to remain in the teaching and learning role. She began to recognize she had an excellent opportunity to advance her education. She had a great desire to earn a doctorate of nursing practice (DNP) degree and began discussing her options with mentors and colleagues. The university in which she was teaching had started a simulation program, and Sandy was involved in that program from the inception. She knew she wanted to incorporate human patient simulation and education into her capstone project.

When conducting literature searches related to simulation and nursing education, Sandy found that medication errors were a recurring theme. The first idea for her proposed capstone project was to implement simulated scenarios into the various nursing courses to decrease medication errors by student nurses and newly graduating novice nurses. That way, the students would be able to use their knowledge and skills in medication administration while causing no harm to live patients. If an error occurred, the students would be able to see the immediate reaction of a medication error.

After having numerous meetings with her faculty advisor and discussing the process for a needs assessment, Sandy completed a needs assessment at the institution. Upon the completion of the needs assessment, it was evident that the institution's faculty were already integrating medication administration in each simulated scenario. Sandy's idea was abandoned because medication administration was already a current practice at the College of Nursing. Additionally, with the guidance of her advisor, Sandy realized the project should have a more inclusive systems-change approach that would be better suited to a hospital setting. A change that could be incorporated into one unit in a hospital had the potential to change the entire culture of education throughout each department within a hospital.

After more meetings with her faculty advisor, Sandy began to explore the practices of area hospitals to determine use of human patient simulation for educational purposes. One area hospital and labor and delivery unit shared a birthing simulator, Noelle, with another area hospital's labor and delivery unit. Each hospital had Noelle to use for a six-month period of time. The labor and delivery nurse educator desperately wanted to utilize the simulator for educational purposes but had no expertise in its application. The nurse educator began explaining that the unit had numerous novice nurses and wanted them to participate in simulated scenarios focused on high-risk, low-volume obstetric patients. Additionally, she commented that The Joint Commission (TJC) would be evaluating the hospital soon and the nursing staff was very weak in knowledge related to the National Patient Safety Goals (NPSG). A shared belief between Sandy and the nurse educator working with the project was that competence in the discipline of nursing is paramount. Maintaining a level of competence is imperative for nursing staff to provide quality and safe patient care. However, competency is challenging to measure due to its many different components. The proposal of annual competencies, including NPSG, was discussed at length with the nurse manager and nurse educator. At this time, buy-in for Sandy's capstone project was obtained.

Further conversations and meetings followed with the unit educator to determine the specific obstetric emergencies and NPSG to be included in the annual competencies. The obstetric emergencies finally selected included fetal distress, amniotic fluid embolism, placental abruption, and postpartum hemorrhage. At the time, 10 NPSG were in existence. Four NPSG were selected for inclusion in the simulated scenarios based on common errors and staff needs: improve the accuracy of patient identification, improve the effectiveness of communication among caregivers, improve the safety of using medications, and accurately and completely reconcile medications across the continuum of care (TJC, 2008).

Sandy then began working closely with her faculty advisor to make the project both meaningful and sustainable. What theory would be the driving force for the project was a question approached first by the advisor. After conducting numerous literature searches and conversations with the faculty advisor, Sandy identified Dr. Patricia Benner's theory, from novice to expert, as the foundation for the project.

At this point, the DNP project had a theoretical basis and needed a model for change. The ACE Star Model of Knowledge Transformation was the model used for the quality improvement project. It enabled the discovery of knowledge to be implemented and transformed into practice. The ACE model consists of five cyclical phases: discovery, summary, translation, integration, and evaluation (Bonis, Taft, & Wender, 2007). While planning and implementing the project of using human patient simulation for annual competency validation for labor and delivery nurses, each phase of the ACE model was encountered.

Many variables were significant in planning for the implementation of each phase of the project. First, the institutional review board (IRB) had to approve the project to maintain protection for those subjects participating in the project. Although the project was one of quality improvement, protection of the participating subjects was an important aspect of the project, including future publication options. Approval by the IRB was required to be obtained before any steps in the implementation phases could begin at the institution. The information provided in the IRB application explained the purpose of the systems change project, as well as the risks and benefits to the participants. The faculty advisor played a major role in assisting and advising Sandy throughout the IRB approval process.

Information throughout the IRB application described the process of implementing the use of human patient simulation for annual competency validation. Although there were no anticipated risks associated with the quality improvement project, there was a minimal risk that staff might experience the normal anxiety typically associated with performance during the annual competency validations. Job security would not be compromised as a result of poor performance during the annual competencies. If the nurses did not perform at a level to meet the goal of 100% compliance, the staff nurse would be provided with review information and given more opportunities to repeat the simulated experience until the desired performance was achieved. However, the projected positive outcome would be an increase in the nursing staff's confidence in their management of obstetric emergencies, especially with high-risk, low-volume patients.

All labor and delivery nurses were required to participate in the annual competencies. Data collected for competency validation were kept confidential.

The successful completion of the annual competencies would be stored in the nurse's personnel folder to maintain confidentiality. However, some level of privacy and confidentiality would be lost due group participation, evaluation, and debriefing.

Approximately 60 labor and delivery nurses participated in the annual competency validation. The anticipated outcomes of the annual competency validations were positive. The goal of 100% compliance was met with each labor and delivery nurse. Human patient simulation provided an excellent learning opportunity for the labor and delivery nurses.

**Continuous quality improvement** was evident throughout the entire systems change process. The project provided benefits to both the hospital staff and their obstetric patients. Because the purpose of the project was one of quality improvement, the Institute of Medicine (IOM) aims were an important factor in the project, although each aim was not distinctly defined in this case. In general, the IOM aims include patient-centeredness, safety, effectiveness, efficiency, timeliness, and equity (Institute for Healthcare Improvement, 2009). Each aim was addressed in Sandy's quality improvement project, but the aim of safety was clearly a focal point throughout the implementation of the project. The project also incorporated evidence supporting human patient simulation as an effective learning tool for staff nurses. Experience is imperative for nurses to develop critical thinking skills and achieve competence. Once critical thinking skills and proficiency of psychomotor skills have been established, patient safety can be ensured.

The component of **sustainability** was in place from the initial meeting with the nurse manager and nurse educator. Many inquiries were made during the project regarding different strategies to incorporate into future simulated experiences for annual competencies. At the completion of the project, educational information and modules for the educator, as well as the staff nurses, were given to the unit educator for future use of the simulator. Information included in the modules dealt with pathophysiology, incidence, assessments, interventions, evidence-based practice articles, and case studies related to each of the obstetrical emergencies. Additionally, general information regarding The Joint Commission, accreditation, National Patient Safety Goals, and elements of performance were included in the nurse's educational module.

Additional training and information were provided for educating the unit educator to maintain the sustainability of the project. Hands-on training, ranging from assembly of the simulator to moulaging to running scenarios, was provided to enable the unit educator to become proficient in using the simulator. A user manual was also developed for the unit educator, which included written and pictorial guides for future use.

Finally, several evaluation tools were developed and used for various aspects of the project and given to the nurse educator. One evaluation tool was developed to evaluate competence for each nurse with the obstetric emergencies as well as the chosen NPSG to be completed by the unit educator. Upon completion of the simulated scenarios, the staff nurses were given another evaluation tool to evaluate the experience during the scenarios.

Because it was well received by the institution and all of those involved, Sandy's project had great potential for sustainability. The labor and delivery unit educator planned to continue to use human patient simulation for annual competency validations. Also, other departments in the hospital were interested in using human patient simulation for various educational needs. One very exciting possibility was interprofessional use of human patient simulation, which was under discussion by the departments. The dissemination of findings, a very important factor, was also guided and supported by the faculty advisor. The project was presented at various conferences and introduced to surrounding hospitals.

The guidance by Sandy's advisor throughout the entire process of the quality improvement project and systems change was critical to the project's success. Without the direction and education provided by the advisor related to evidence, the project's theoretical basis, the project plan, the IRB process, analysis of data, and dissemination of the results, the project would not have had a solid foundation or the ability to maintain sustainability. Incorporating the use of human patient simulation for annual competency validation in a labor and delivery unit was a process that encompassed multiple strategic methods and various models. Obstetric emergencies are rare occurrences, but the nursing staff must be competent and maintain the ability to respond to them quickly and appropriately. The advisor, Sandy, the nurse educator, and the nurse manager firmly supported the use of human patient simulation for annual competency validation. The simulated scenarios assisted in bridging the gap between real patients and the learning opportunities for the labor and delivery nursing staff. Additionally, the incorporation of the National Patient Safety Goals into the simulated experiences assisted the organizations in maintaining compliance with The Joint Commission standards.

## Reflection Questions

1.  What are the benefits of completing a needs assessment prior to developing a clinical project? Consider which parts of a needs assessment may benefit you later as you engage in a clinical project.
2.  How might a faculty advisor guide students throughout the clinical project?
3.  How does completing the IRB process benefit the clinical project and its sustainability?

## References

Bonis, S., Taft, L. & Wender, C. (2007). Strategies to promote success on the NCLEX-RN: An evidence-based approach using the ACE star model of knowledge transformation [Electronic version]. *Nursing Education Perspectives, 2*, 82–87.

Institute for Healthcare Improvement. (2009). Science of improvement: setting aims. http://www .ihi.org/resources/Pages/HowtoImprove/ScienceofImprovementSettingAims.aspx

The Joint Commission (TJC). (2008). National patient safety goals. http://www.jointcommission.org

# ■ CASE STUDY 2

## Praxis: The Benefit to the Chief Nursing Officer as Projects Are Planned and Implemented

*Frank Garrison*

In any professional discipline, the overarching question of what guides practice is essential to understanding the framework within which practice occurs (Cody, 2013). Many factors influence the integration of theories and experiences that form the practice choices of an individual, and understanding the interrelation of those factors allows the individual to pursue knowledge, articulate practice, and communicate ideas more effectively. The process of integrating those theories and experiences is the underlying concept of praxis. As explained by Rolfe (1993), praxis is an ongoing, circular process of reflection in action whereby theory and practice continually inform, modify, and guide each other. Understanding the integration of informal theory and practice, a nurse executive can advance the profession and improve practice through a continual, circular process of reflection and action as projects are planned, implemented, and evaluated.

As the healthcare industry is evolving into a more technology-driven and resource-limited business model, the role of the nurse executive is becoming more business-focused. Certainly, clinical knowledge and skill are required for effective leadership of a nursing workforce, but a nurse executive also must understand how to direct quality care efficiently and communicate and collaborate effectively. Nurse executives must lead quality improvement initiatives to ensure cost-effective delivery of quality care (Carlson & Staffileno, 2014). Using relevant influences to form a nursing praxis to guide leadership allows for a structured, intentional approach to practice. By intentionally operating within the framework of a personal praxis, a nurse executive will continually improve leadership and advance the profession as projects evolve.

## Ideological, Theoretical, and Ethical Influences

For a chief nursing officer, embracing an analytic approach as the primary philosophical viewpoint for practice allows for quantifying and measuring a variety of operational metrics. Based on empiricism, an analytic approach involves quantifiable data and definable results (Monti & Tingen, 1999). Empirical data allow a chief nursing officer to analyze relationships between quality improvement measures and cost savings strategies. However, incorporating the continental approach to understand qualitative factors also is important for addressing less quantifiable aspects of nursing care and leadership (Monti & Tingen, 1999). Integrating both the analytic and continental approaches into leadership practice provides for a greater understanding of the nursing meta-paradigm and other relevant theoretical influences that guide projects throughout all phases.

From the broader framework of Fawcett's (1984) nursing meta-paradigm, Orem's (1991) Self-Care Deficit Nursing Theory (SCDNT) acts as instructive guide for teaching organizational goals for improving patient health and decreasing readmissions. McMahon and Christopher's (2011) middle-range theory for teaching the aesthetic skill of nursing presence also is an excellent guide for continued education of nurses. In addition to nursing theories, the field of complexity science offers important guidance for practice in the explanation and understanding of complex adaptive systems. Chief nursing officers must recognize the potential butterfly effect when even a small project or practice change is implemented (Florczak, Poradzisz, & Hampson, 2012).

Operating within an ethical framework also is imperative to effective and professional nursing practice. The theory of virtue ethics offers an appropriate context for professional practice. Focusing on the qualities of compassion, discernment, trustworthiness, integrity, and conscientiousness, virtue ethics provides a guideline for developing the qualities necessary for professionalism and for integrating those qualities into practice (Chism, 2013). In any leadership activity, a chief nursing officer must recognize the importance of instilling in nurses the ethical standards required for practice. By integrating the virtue ethics framework with the hospital-specific code of ethics, a nurse executive can communicate effectively to the nursing workforce the ethical expectations for practice. Keeping in mind the relevance of an ethics framework and its transparency is also pivotal as any project transpires.

Figure 1-1    Chief Nursing Officer framework for praxis.

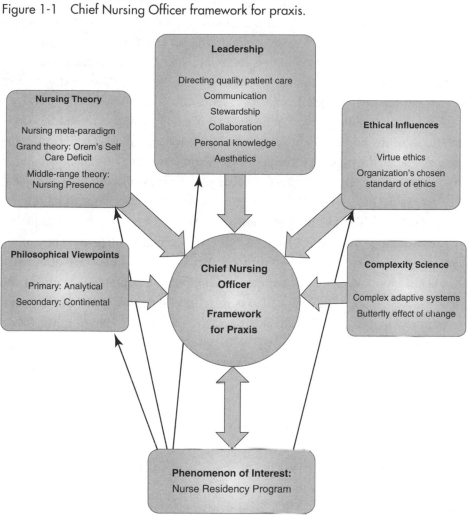

## Utilization of Framework: A Case Study

Understanding the benefit of a nursing praxis can be demonstrated by analyzing a chief nursing officer's (CNO) personal praxis (**Figure 1-1**) in the context of the phenomenon of interest of nurse residency programs (NRPs) for new gradu- ate registered nurses (RNs). Analyzing empirical data related to a high level of

RN vacancies across the hospital, the CNO quantified the operational impact of the vacancies. Hospital volume was increasing, but the size of the RN workforce remained stagnant. Hospital policy required any RN being hired to have at least two years of RN experience. Available qualitative information revealed engagement and organizational loyalty within the existing RN workforce were decreasing due to the work demands caused by the vacancies.

Understanding the ethical obligation to provide quality care and the stewardship responsibilities for leading nursing practice, the CNO discerned the need to change the policy on hiring only experienced RNs. This change required implementing a NRP to address the needs of RNs transitioning to professional practice. In designing the NRP, the CNO stressed the importance of communicating the SCDNT for health promotion and the use of nursing presence theory to guide training simulations. Understanding the complex, adaptive nature of the hospital, the CNO anticipated a positive butterfly effect as the NRP eliminated vacancies, increased RN engagement, and improved the quality of care. As the NRP proceeded, the CNO planned to collect data on the effects of the NRP and determine which data will influence the CNO's praxis (Figure 1-1) for future guidance.

## Reflection Questions

1. What are two benefits of praxis to nurses assigned to clinical and administrative roles?
2. How can you use the benefits of praxis to enhance your nursing knowledge and practice?

## References

Carlson, E. A., & Staffileno, B. A. (2013). Establishing and sustaining an evidence-based practice environment. In M. A. Mateo & M. D. Foreman (Eds.), *Research for advanced practice nurses, from evidence to practice* (2nd ed.), 69–86. New York, NY: Springer.
Chism, L. A. (2013). The DNP graduate as ethical consultant. In L. A. Chism (Ed.), *The doctor of nursing practice* (2nd ed.), 179–212. Burlington, MA: Jones & Bartlett Learning.

Cody, W. K. (2013). Values-based practice and evidence-based care: Pursing fundamental questions in nursing philosophy and theory. In W. K. Cody (Ed.), *Philosophical and theoretical perspectives for advanced nursing practice* (5th ed.), 5–13. Burlington, MA: Jones & Bartlett Learning.

Fawcett, J. (1984). The meta-paradigm of nursing: Current status and future refinements. *Image: Journal of Nursing Scholarship, 16*, 84–87. http://www.nursingsociety.org/Publication

Florczak, K., Poradzisz, M., & Hampson, S. (2012). Nursing in a complex world: A case for grand theory. *Nursing Science Quarterly, 25*, 307–312. doi: 10.1177/0894318412457069

McMahon, M. A., & Christopher, K. A. (2011). Toward a mid-range theory of nursing presence. *Nursing Forum, 46*, 72–82. doi: 10.1111/j.1744-6198.2011.00215.x

Monti, E. J., & Tingen, M. S. (1999). Multiple paradigms of nursing science. *Advances in Nursing Science, 21*, 64–80. http://journals.lww.com/advancesinnursingscience/pages/default.aspx

Orem, D. E. (1991). *Nursing: Concepts of practice* (4th ed.). St. Louis, MO: Mosby.

Rolfe, G. (1993). Closing the theory-practice gap: A model of nursing praxis. *Journal of Clinical Nursing, 2*, 173–177. doi: 10.1111/j.1365-2702.1993.tb00157.x

## CHAPTER TWO

# Differentiating Quality Improvement Projects and Quality Improvement Research

*Linda Roussel*

## Chapter Objectives

1. Define quality improvement and the primary elements.
2. Differentiate between quality improvement projects and quality improvement research.
3. List considerations related to implementation science, translational science, and dissemination of both quality improvement projects and quality improvement research.

## Key Terms

| | | |
|---|---|---|
| Innovation | Quality improvement | Value |
| Project planning | | |

## Roles

| | |
|---|---|
| Advocate | Leader |

## Professional Values

| | | |
|---|---|---|
| Evidence-based practice | Patient-centered care | Quality |

## Core Competencies

| | | |
|---|---|---|
| Assessment | Design | Management |
| Coordination | Leadership | Risk mitigation |

## Introduction

The Health Resources and Services Administration (HRSA, 2011) defines **quality improvement** as a systematic and continuous process that leads to measurable improvement in healthcare services and the health status of a targeted patient population. As a process for improving quality outcomes, strategies are employed in an intentional way to assure that there is flow from the gaps (needs assessment) to the planning, implementing, and evaluation phases. The Institute of Medicine (IOM, 2001) defines quality in health care as a direct relationship between the level of improved health services and the expected health outcomes of individuals and populations. Quality improvement strategies are integral to projects that focus on safety, improvement, and **innovation**. Understanding of the basic principles of quality improvement and quality improvement research is the cornerstone of projects that are impactful and add **value**.

This chapter seeks to define quality improvement and identify the primary elements in the quality improvement cycle. How quality improvement projects and quality improvement research are differentiated is described as well. In addition, this chapter considers related improvement sciences, such as translational and implementation science.

## Quality Improvement

Quality improvement requires thoughtful leadership in nursing as a major driver in advancing positive healthcare outcomes. Shewhart (1931) first studied quality from an industrial perspective, which led him to introduce concepts such as customer needs, reduction in variations in process, and elimination of the need for frequent inspections. Intrigued by Shewhart's work, Deming (1982) was able to determine that quality was a major driver for positive outcomes in industry; in turn, he introduced quality methodology to post–World War II Japanese engineers and executives. Deming's methods were strategically applied by the Japanese automobile industry, which enabled members of this industry— and other Japanese industries —to gain worldwide recognition for the quality of their products and services (Deming, 1982). Shewhart's and Deming's work on quality control has since informed the work of the Institute for Healthcare Improvement (IHI) and the Model for Improvement (MFI). The MFI is considered foundational to many of the quality models, such as Six Sigma, Lean Toyota, and the define–measure–analyze–improve–control (DMAIC) process (IHI, 2015a).

From the IOM's perspective, quality is considered within an organization's current system and is defined as how work gets done. Healthcare performance, however, is defined based on the organization's efficiency, care outcomes, and patient satisfaction levels. Quality is directly aligned with an organization's service delivery approach or underlying systems of care. Innovation is necessary to achieve a different level of performance and improve quality. From a **project planning** and management perspective on improving quality, it is important to understand the principles underpinning quality initiatives. The IOM purports that while a quality project may be unique to the organization, all successful quality initiatives integrate four key principles:

1.  Quality improvement work as systems and processes
2.  Focus on patients
3.  Focus on being part of the team
4.  Focus on use of the data

## Quality Improvement as Systems and Processes

If an organization is to make improvements, understanding its own delivery system and key processes are critical to beginning this work. Quality improvement approaches recognize available resources (inputs) and tasks carried out (processes), which collectively determine quality of care (outputs/outcomes). For example, inputs may include people, infrastructure, materials, information, and technology. Consideration is given to the professionals and providers within the system, as well as to the supplies and equipment needed to carry out the project.

Processes involve activities focusing on what is to be done and how the project will be carried out. Consequently, process-flow maps and concept maps are useful tools in illustrating the steps in carrying out the work. The process map, which comes to health care from engineering, provides a visual diagram that chronicles events or steps culminating in particular outcomes. The visualization of those steps provides a concrete look at how the work (processes) is carried out, as well as who is accountable for that work and how efficiently the work flows, and can illuminate areas for improvement. Knowledge of how work flows may indicate the need for redesign, and the proposed plan can be compared to previous processes that are not working. Tools and resources to assist in developing projects using process mapping as an improvement strategy can be found at the Institute for Healthcare

Improvement's website: http://www.ihi.org/education/WebTraining/OnDe mand/Pages/default.aspx.

Gaps in the process can lead to further explorations, such as through failure model effect analysis (FMEA). FMEA is a tool used for risk mitigation, which is essential to achieving safe, quality outcomes (IHI, 2015b). This type of analysis requires that each step (or process) be assessed for severity and frequency, with a hazard score being constructed to summarize these results. High hazard scores (8 or greater) alert the improvement team that emergent action is needed, particularly when the processes involve more than a single point, have few or no controls, and are not detectable (IHI, 2015c).

Outputs or outcomes may consider results or patterns such as health services delivered, changes in health behaviors and health status, and patient satisfaction. Health service delivery systems may be small, simple, and straightforward, such as a well-baby clinic, or multilayered and complex, such as a large corporate proprietary system. The efficiency and efficacy of the system depend on the services being individualized and attending to specific needs within the system. When the system considers the resources, activities, and results that exist and that are desired, quality improvement projects and programs can be customized to address unmet needs.

## Focus on Patients

Patient-centered care is not a new concept; indeed, it has been reinforced as a competency for educating healthcare professionals in the 21st century (IOM, 2001). Patient-centered care evolved with resurgence of the holistic roots of health care, and initially had limited appeal given the complexity of the present healthcare system. Defined as engaging patients in a true partnership, patient-centered care involves personalizing care to include patients' normal routines and values. Such aims were considered daunting objectives when first introduced, and unrealistic at best. With increased technology and patient involvement, however, the creation of a healing physical environment, including one in which spiritual and emotional needs are met, has become mainstream practice.

So important is patient-centered care that the Hospital Consumer Assessment of Healthcare Providers and Systems (HCAHPS) created a patient survey that affords patients the opportunity to share information about their experiences with the healthcare system. In other words, this standardized tool assesses the way care is provided from the patients' perspective. Considering care from the patients' perspective takes into account more than just clinical treatment, medications, and technology. While core measures provide data that evaluate hospitals' care quality, at a minimum from a standard of care perspective, the patient experience is not necessarily taken into consideration when evaluating overall care delivery. HCAHPS considers aspects of the healthcare experience that patients report are important to them on a personal level, such as communication with nurses and physicians, cleanliness and noise levels, pain control, and quality of discharge instructions and medication information. Publicly reported scores of individual hospital systems have health systems on high alert, given that patients can now compare the way care is delivered by various system and decide which is the best fit for them as individuals. With the advent of value-based purchasing, HCAHPS data have become increasingly important as a basis for reimbursement, further informing and advancing patient-centered care. Responding to these demands by delivering patient-centered care has also become an important business imperative.

The healthcare system's focus on patients is an important measure of quality that considers the patients' needs and expectations. When a focus on patients is present, services are created and designed by paying attention to the following factors: systems that affect patient access; care provision that is evidence-based; patient safety; support for patient engagement; coordination of care with other parts of the larger healthcare system; and cultural competence, including assessing health literacy of patients, patient-centered communication, and linguistically appropriate care (HRSA, 2011).

## Focus on Being Part of the Team

Quality improvement (QI) is a "team sport." QI as a team process denotes the importance of the team coming together to take advantage of the knowledge, skills, experience, and perspectives of individual providers and professionals within the team to make sustainable improvements and produce innovations. Team effectiveness can happen when the following elements are in play: considering the process or system as complex; acknowledging that no one person in an organization knows all the dimensions of an issue; recognizing that the process involves more than one discipline or work area; advocating for solutions that require creativity; and realizing that staff commitment and buy-in are needed. All QI projects engage individuals as part of a team and implement QI as a team process. Projects such as improving time to referring providers, increasing patient engagement, reducing wait time, and ensuring providers' use of evidence-based guidelines are team efforts that can go far toward achieving sustainable improvements. Active involvement of team members is critical, as each individual skill set and contribution leads to a synthesis and synergy of ideas and solutions that would not have the same impact if they were implemented in isolation.

Another key component of a well-organized and functioning QI team is an effective infrastructure, such as leadership and policies/procedures that design and facilitate the work of the team. A strong infrastructure provides the team with tools, resources, clarity of expectations, and a medium for communication (HRSA, 2011).

## Focus on the Use of Data

A centerpiece of QI is the use of data. Data can be used to determine how effectively current systems are working and what occurs when changes are applied, and to document successful performance. By using data, the team is able to accomplish a number of tasks. First, the QI team members are able to separate what they believe is happening from what is actually happening within the system. A baseline can then be established to determine which, if any, changes made would be an improvement. It is likely that baseline scores will be low (this is acceptable), so the aim is to improve the rates and scores (e.g., patient satisfaction, falls, pressure ulcers, wait times, restraint use). By tracking data and comparing the baseline to the post-intervention data, the team can determine the efficacy of solutions; likewise, by monitoring procedural changes, it can evaluate whether improvements are sustained over time. In this way, data serve as powerful sources by which to determine whether the changes made led to improvements, and they allow for comparisons of performance across sites.

Quantitative and qualitative methods of collecting data are essential to QI projects. The use of numbers (rates, scores) and frequencies represents a quantitative research method that results in measurable data. Statistical process control, for instance, provides a wealth of information that can measure efficiency in care delivery. Examples include calculating how frequently patients access the emergency room and receive adequate health screenings. While numbers, rates, and frequency provide excellent ways to measure improvement efforts, the use of qualitative methods sheds light on the depth and breadth of the experience of care delivery. Data that are qualitative in nature are observable (not measurable), consider patterns and relationships between systems, and are contextual in nature. Qualitative methods may include patient and staff satisfaction surveys, focus groups, interviews, and participant-observation experiences.

Healthcare organizations can obtain data from a number of sources, including health records, patient and staff satisfaction surveys, external evaluations from accrediting and regulatory agencies, and community assessments. Using data sources in a methodical way within the infrastructure of an organizational system illuminates opportunities for improvement and allows for ongoing monitoring. Standardized performance measures focus on specific data for QI programs. Healthcare organizations are encouraged to collect data on performance measures that are impactful and add value to both the patient experience and the overall operation of the healthcare system. Such outcomes should guide the organizations' decisions regarding which data are collected and measured.

## Quality Improvement Programs and Quality Improvement Research

With a QI program, the QI team considers the systematic activities that are designed and implemented to monitor, assess, and improve the organization's quality of health care for the population it serves. Higher levels of performance are reflected upon when reviewing the cyclical activities that are implemented to optimize resources and services for the patients served. There is a creative tension between innovation, sustained improvement, and ongoing delivery of evidence-based standards of care. Organizational QI programs incorporate all QI activities within the healthcare system.

The Donabedian model of structure, process, and outcomes provides a theoretical framework for integrating quality improvement strategies within the system (Donabedian, 1988). Leadership and interdisciplinary teams are essential to sustained quality improvement programs. Likewise, knowledge of the infrastructure and the principles of quality improvement is foundational to a successful QI program. Leaders ask the question of how QI processes work to support the success of the QI program. A number of benefits can be achieved from implementing a QI program, including improved patient (clinical) outcomes that focus on process outcomes (screenings) and health outcomes (blood glucose and blood pressure readings within normal parameters). Other benefits of QI programs are improved efficiency of managerial and clinical processes, such as reducing waste and maintaining financial viability.

According to HRSA, by improving processes and outcomes that reflect high-priority health needs, a system is able to reduce costs associated with system failures and redundancy. QI processes are typically budget-neutral, meaning that the costs incurred to make the changes are offset by the savings obtained through those efforts. QI programs put proactive processes in place and solve problems before they occur, making sure that systems of care are consistent, reliable, and predictable. These actions can go far in creating a culture of improvement, as they ensure that errors are tracked, reported, and addressed. Critical issues are often resolved because greater attention is paid to monitoring improvement initiatives and variations in standards of care. With a culture of improvement in place, communication is enhanced both within the system and among community organizations. Improved communication focused on quality may result in stronger clinical partnerships and open up funding opportunities. An effective QI program can result in a balance of quality, efficiency, and profitability in its achievement of organizational goals (HRSA, 2011).

## Quality Improvement Research

QI projects may come under the federal definition of research, and may require institutional review board (IRB) review and approval if they involve human participants or individually identifiable data. QI programs and QI research should not pose any risk to individuals, infringe on individual privacy, or breach individual confidentiality (*Institutional Review Board Guidebook*, 2015). Research in this context is defined as follows:

> 45 CFR 46.102(d) of the federal regulations defines research as a systematic investigation, including research development, testing and evaluation designed to develop or contribute to generalizable knowledge.

One characteristic that distinguishes a QI program from QI research is whether the activities are intended or created to develop or contribute to generalizable knowledge. Results or research findings, when they are generalizable knowledge, can be applied to populations or situations beyond those being immediately studied. When quality improvement initiatives are not intended to yield generalizable knowledge, IRB review is not mandatory.

In contrast, QI research that is planned in advance to go beyond the scope of the unit, department, or services would require IRB approval. For example, the QI team may want the results from its analysis and the interpretation of its quality initiative to be disseminated across a larger scope and to a broader community of scholars. In other cases, quality improvement research may be intended for application beyond the current quality control efforts or improvements, as when new procedures or processes are shared with a larger audience (outside of one system).

If at least one of these descriptions of QI research applies to the team's QI plan, the next consideration would be whether the proposed activities and strategies are a systematic investigation. When applying the concept of systematic investigation, the team would determine whether information beyond what is routine for patient care will be collected. For example, adding surveys or more data collection through qualitative means, which is typically not part of routine care delivery, would go beyond a QI program. Another consideration with a systematic investigation would be to determine if the team will be assessing the effectiveness or processes or procedures and comparing two or more treatments, interventions, or processes. When such comparison is contemplated, and manipulation is done to determine if one practice is better, the effort would qualify as QI research. When QI activities entail a systematic investigation that will develop or contribute to generalizable knowledge, per 45 CFR 46.102(d), IRB review is mandatory.

At the outset, many QI projects have only local (organizational) assurance/improvement intentions; during the process of data collection or analysis, however, it may become clear that the findings could be generalizable or benefit others. In such a case, IRB review should occur—that is, IRB review is necessary whenever there is an intention to make findings generalizable.

## Quality Improvement and Beyond

While nurses are the largest subgroup in the healthcare system, they lack representation on decision-making bodies. QI activities can increase nurses' influence and involvement in decision making at the policy level. A Gallup survey conducted by the Robert Wood Johnson Foundation, titled "Nursing Leadership from the Bedside to the Boardroom: Opinion Leaders' Perception" (Gallup/Robert Wood Johnson Foundation, 2010), reported that the persons surveyed considered government executives (75%) and health insurance executives (56%) as being able to exert more influence on health reform than nurses, whom they ranked as having only 14% influence (Khoury, Blizzard, Moore, & Hassmiller, 2011). These numbers demonstrate that nurses, especially those in positions of authority, need to encourage the development of leaders within the profession and advocate for interprofessional QI team activity. Quality improvement programs provide an excellent opportunity for nurses to become involved in sustainable changes and policy development.

Beyond QI's immediate impact and results, consideration should be given to dissemination of both QI projects and QI research. Translational science, including improvement and implementation sciences, is also important to developing QI science.

Healthcare providers and consumers of health care are becoming more aware that research results that may have broad application do not always readily translate into improved health outcomes. The implementation and dissemination of research and science rely on a multidisciplinary set of theories and methods aimed at improving this process of translation from research evidence to pragmatic health-related practices. Implementation research, in particular, investigates how interventions can best be integrated into diverse practice settings and underscores direct engagement with the institutions and communities where health interventions are introduced. Team science and organizational and cultural perspectives are also integrated into translational science, as the gold standard of research (randomized controlled trials) often does not take into account the details necessary for application of findings.

Disseminating QI projects and research can take many forms, such as local stakeholder engagement; poster and podium presentations at regional, national, and international venues; and publication of manuscripts that share findings obtained, barriers overcome, and lessons learned. An excellent resource for dissemination of results is the Agency for Healthcare Research and Quality's (AHRQ) Health Care Innovations Exchange (https://innovations.ahrq.gov). The Innovation Exchange is a web-based resource created to assist healthcare professionals in sharing and adopting innovations that improve healthcare quality. The website includes a clearinghouse of innovative ideas and opportunities to learn and share ideas with others.

Using research evidence to develop evidence-based practice guidelines is also important in the application and translation process of QI projects and research. The National Guidelines Clearinghouse (NGC) is another initiative of the Agency for Healthcare Research and Quality. It was originally created by AHRQ in partnership with the American Medical Association and the American Association of Health Plans (now America's Health Insurance Plans [AHIP]). The mission of the NGC is "to provide health professionals, healthcare providers, health plans, integrated delivery systems, purchasers, and others with a readily usable mechanism for accessing objective, detailed information on clinical practice guidelines and to further their dissemination, implementation, and use" (http://www.guideline.gov/about/index.aspx).

QI projects and research can also be disseminated through manuscript submissions. A useful tool in writing up QI projects is the Standards for Quality

Improvement Reporting Excellence (SQUIRE) guidelines. According to its sponsoring organization (http://squire-statement.org/), the SQUIRE guidelines assist authors in writing up excellent, usable articles about quality improvement in health care. The guidelines serve as a way to report findings that may be easily discovered and widely disseminated. The SQUIRE website notes that high-quality writing about improvement, lists of available resources, and discussions about the writing process can enhance dissemination and adoption of best practices. Sponsors of the SQUIRE guidelines include the Dartmouth Institute for Health Policy and Clinical Practice, the Robert Wood Johnson Foundation, Quality and Safety in Healthcare, and the Institute for Healthcare Improvement.

QI projects and research can also be shared through the Honor Society of Nursing, Sigma Theta Tau International. Its e-Repository hosts communities and collections that can be accessed and applied in practice, as well as a method of disseminating quality projects and research. According to the website, the Henderson Repository, a resource of Sigma Theta Tau International, offers the following benefits:

- *Online dissemination.* This global digital service collects, preserves, and shares nursing research and evidence-based practice materials.
- *Free open access.* There is no charge to submitting nurse authors and no access fee for online patrons.
- *Peer review.* Submissions to collections under the Independent Submissions community are peer reviewed (http://www.nursinglibrary.org/vhl/).

Dissemination of evidence and information takes many forms, and methods for quality improvement and quality improvement research can be shared with many colleagues through these means. Evidence-based journal clubs and clinical scholars programs are other ways to raise the level of conversation, create a spirit of inquiry, and enhance the culture of improvement in health care.

## Summary

- Quality improvement projects and quality improvement research share common aims for making healthcare systems safe and quality-driven.

- Leading a quality team that is focused on patient-centered care and using data to inform the process are essential to the work of clinical nurse leaders, executive leadership students, doctors of nursing practice (DNP), and highly functioning interprofessional project teams.
- The foundational work for the development of quality improvement projects and research is key to sustaining success over the long term.

## Reflection Questions

1. Describe quality improvement projects you are currently involved in as part of your practice immersion experience.
2. Access the AHRB Innovation Exchange, and select an innovation that best aligns with your quality improvement work. How you are able to use the evidence and strategies described for the innovation?
3. Access the National Clearinghouse Guidelines (NCG). Which guideline can you adopt in providing evidence-based care with your own patient populations?

## References

Agency for Healthcare for Research and Quality. (n.d.). Innovation Exchange. https://innovations.ahrq.gov

Deming, E. W. (1982). *Out of crisis.* Cambridge, MA: MIT Center for Advanced Engineering Study.

Donabedian, A. (1988). The quality of care: How can it be assessed? *Journal of the American Medical Association, 260*(12), 1743–1748. doi: 10.1001/jama.1988.03410120089033

Gallup/Robert Wood Johnson Foundation. (2010). Nursing leadership from bedside to boardroom: Opinion leaders' perceptions. http://www.rwjf.org/content/dam/web-assets/2010/01/nursing-leadership-from-bedside-to-boardroom

Health Resources and Services Administration (HRSA). (2011). Quality improvement. http://www.hrsa.gov/quality/toolbox/methodology/qualityimprovement/

Institute for Healthcare Improvement (IHI). (2015a). The breakthrough series: IHI's collaborative model for achieving breakthrough improvement. http://www.ihi.org/resources/Pages/IHIWhitePapers/TheBreakthroughSeriesIHIsCollaborativeModelforAchievingBreakthroughImprovement.aspx

Institute for Healthcare Improvement (IHI). (2015b). Failure mode effect analysis tool. http://www.ihi.org/resources/Pages/Tools/FailureModesandEffectsAnalysisTool.aspx

Institute for Healthcare Improvement (IHI). (2015c). How to improve. http://www.ihi.org/resources/Pages/HowtoImprove/default.aspx

Institute of Medicine (IOM), Committee on Quality Health Care in America. (2001). *Crossing the quality chasm: A new health system for the 21st century.* Washington, DC: National Academy Press. http://www.iom.edu/About IOM.aspx

Institutional review board guidebook. (2015). http://www.hhs.gov/ohrp/archive/irb/irb_chapter1.htm

Khoury, C. M., Blizzard, R., Moore, L. W., & Hassmiller, S. (2011). Nursing leadership from bedside to boardroom: A Gallup national survey of opinion leaders. *Journal of Nursing Administration, 41*(7/8), 299–305

National Clearinghouse Guidelines (NCG). (2015). http://www.guideline.gov/about/index.aspx

Shewhart, W. A. (1931). *Economic control of quality of manufactured product.* New York, NY: D. Van Nostrand.

Sigma Theta Tau International, Virginia Henderson Global Nursing e-Repository. (n.d.). http://www.nursinglibrary.org/vhl/

Standards for Quality Improvement Reporting Excellence (SQUIRE). (n.d.). http://squire-statement.org/

# Case Exemplar

## ■ CASE STUDY 1

### Quality Teams Approach to Discharge Planning

*Terri Poe*

A team of doctor of nursing practice (DNP) students engaged their quality team at their practice site to improve discharge planning by reducing non-value-added activities. The students, working together as a team of acute care nurse practitioners (ACNPs), noted a pattern of increasingly long waits for patients to be transferred to another level of care. To confirm that the pattern they experienced was a "true gap," they engaged their team members, the quality committee, and the chief nurse executive (CNE) to share their concerns. To obtain data to examine the outcomes, they were required to submit a question and begin a search of the external evidence. Through their translational courses, the students were able to step through the quality improvement process, beginning with obtaining internal data through a microsystems analysis and a failure mode effect analysis (FMEA), identifying a gap, searching for external evidence (synthesizing the research), and working with the Model for Improvement to begin small test of change. As they progressed in their quality improvement work, they were able to bring team members along by charting a team, examining the process (through a process flow map), and using plan–do–study–act (PDSA) as a methodological framework for their scholarly project.

## Reflection Questions

1.  How can faculty best assure that doctoral students and interprofessional teams consistently go through a quality improvement process in which they will be able to engage their local stakeholders?
2.  After completing the first iteration of the PDSA method, what would you suggest is the best way for doctoral students and teams to disseminate their results from the first cycle?

## ■ CASE STUDY 2

### Action Plans as an Effective Asthma Management Tool: A Proposed Quality Improvement Project

*Heather Surcouf*

Asthma affects more than 22 million Americans. Asthma exacerbations lead to missed school, low quality of life, missed days on the job, hospitalizations, and emergency room visits. Multiple studies support asthma action plans (AAPs) as effective tools for asthma management.

At one school-based health center in Louisiana, the AAP completion rates declined markedly after adoption of an electronic health record (EHR). A project utilizing electronic health record reminders to prompt providers to complete asthma action plans has been proposed. These reminders will be set to "pop up" in the EHR when an AAP is due. The provider will have to record which action is taken (e.g., AAP completed, rescheduled, cancelled) to move beyond this pop-up. These reminders will automatically reset to appear on a yearly basis. The project relies on the Donabedian Model of Quality Care for theoretical structure. The Deming cycle and plan–do–study–act (PDSA) method of quality monitoring will also be used to assure continued quality improvements.

Specific project goals include the following: (1) increased provider AAP completion rates, (2) continued Office of Public Health clinic funding secondary to AAP benchmark satisfaction, and (3) reduced asthma exacerbation–related clinic visits. Congruent with the guidelines of the American Association of Colleges of Nursing (AACN), and advanced nursing practice (DNP Essentials), this project will evaluate provider use of information systems and technology to support and improve patient care using the AAP (AACN, 2006, p.12).

Records of patients with asthma (ages 14–21) will be audited both before and after project implementation for the presence of a completed, up-to-date asthma action plan. Pre-implementation data and post-implementation data for two separate 9-month periods will be compiled through a retrospective review of the electronic records of patients seen in the clinic for a 9-month period prior to the study and for a 9-month period after the study's implementation, based on their diagnosis of asthma (ICD-9 codes 493.00 to 493.92). Records included for review will be determined through the electronic record's reporting program. Results will be tabulated using a frequency table (i.e., the number of patients with asthma with a completed AAP and the number of patients with asthma without a completed AAP). A second frequency table will be used to tally the number of asthma-related visits for the same study periods using identical ICD-9 codes. Lastly, providers will be given an anonymous survey before and after the intervention to gauge their familiarity with EHR reminders as well as their opinion regarding their effectiveness.

## Reflection Questions

1. What is the value of an action plan in managing clinical symptoms?
2. How can medical record reminders promote patient-centered care delivery?
3. Identify tools that are useful in implementing quality improvement projects. Which of the tools are most useful when developing and implementing projects?

## References

Bell, L. M., Grundmeier, R., Localio, R., Zorc, J., Fiks, A. G., Zhang, X., . . . Guevara, J. P. (2010). Electronic health record-based decision support to improve asthma care: A cluster-randomized trial. *Pediatrics, 125*(4), e770–e774. doi: 10.1542/peds.2009-1385

Centers for Disease Control and Management. (2007, May 4). CDC vital signs: Asthma in the U.S. http://www.cdc.gov/vitalsigns/asthma/

Ducharme, F. M., & Bhogal, S. K. (2008). The role of written action plans in childhood asthma. *Current Opinion in Allergy and Clinical Immunology, 8*(2), 177–188. http://www.ncbi.nlm.nih.gov/pmc/articles/PMC3522127/

Halterman, J. S., Fisher, S., Conn, K. S., Fagnano, M., Lynch, K., Marky, A., & Szilagyi, P. G. (2006). Improved preventive care for asthma: A randomized trial of clinician prompting in pediatric offices. *Archives of Pediatrics and Adolescent Medicine, 160*, 1018–1025. http://archpedi.jamanetwork.com; links.com/index.php

Tolomeo, C., Shiffman, R., & Bazzy-Asaad, A. (2008). Electronic medical records in a subspecialty practice: One asthma center's experience. *Journal of Asthma, 45*(9), 849–851. doi: 10.1080/02770900802380803

Turkelson, C., & Hughes, J.E. (2006). Why aren't you doing evidence based practice? [Reprint]. *AAOS Bulletin, 54*(3), 1–4. http://www5.aaos.org/oko/ebp/EBP001/suppPDFs/OKO_EBP001_S23.pdf

## CHAPTER THREE

# The Institutional Review Board Process

*Catherine Dearman, Jennifer Styron,
and Sheila Whitworth*

## *Chapter Objectives*

1.  Examine the process for initiating and completing the institutional review board (IRB) process—the when, why, and how to navigate the process.
2.  Formulate a crosswalk that features the parts associated with initiating and completing the IRB process.

## *Key Terms*

Human subject
  protection
Human subjects

Informed consent
Institutional review
  board (IRB)

## *Roles*

Participant

Researcher

Reviewer

## *Professional Values*

Beneficence
Quality

Respect for persons
Social justice

## *Core Competencies*

Analysis
Communication

Design
Development

# Introduction

This chapter reviews the role of the **institutional review board (IRB)** in an organization and describes the basic process used in the review of a study. The institutional review board is integral to the protection of **human subjects** and connecting those subjects to the protocols and safeguards included in completing an IRB application. Organizations sponsoring research and other scholarly work must consider the impact of that work on human subjects and be able to determine whether information gleaned from the work can be generalized to the public. Therefore, IRB approval should be secured prior to any data collection for research and quality improvement projects.

The IRB comprises a representative group of faculty and staff within an institution who are experienced in research processes and thoroughly understand how the rights of subjects in the research are protected. The IRB reviews all research and many quality improvement protocols involving human subjects prior to their implementation, to assure that subjects' human rights are protected. In many cases, IRB approval is a basic requirement to publication of the findings, including those from quality improvement projects.

Inherent in the IRB review is the independent nature of the review and the reviewers—that is, researchers do not review their own work, but rather independent members of the IRB review each submission. In some cases, more than one IRB will need to be involved in the review of the research, especially if the university is not connected to the clinical facility where the research will occur.

Regardless of the project that is identified, the initial step is to complete a needs assessment, analyze the data, and assimilate data as background support when building the business case. However, one cannot dismiss the need to obtain IRB approval if the data or outcomes of a project will be disseminated beyond the immediate organization or system. Securing IRB approval at the beginning of the project limits future issues.

## Historical Perspective Related to Protection of Human Subjects

The Federal Policy for the Protection of Human Subjects requires universities or other institutions that receive federal funds and conduct biomedical or behavioral research involving human subjects to establish an institutional review process. The "Common Rule," as the policy is widely known, requires a research institution to assure the protection of the human rights of human subjects who participate in research. The institution is bound by law, then, to assure that all researchers follow this rule with regard to selecting subjects and obtaining

**informed consent** from them (U.S. Department of Health and Human Services [DHHS], 2011, 2012).

IRBs emerged based on principles included in the Nuremberg Code, the Declaration of Helsinki (World Medical Association, 2008), and the Belmont Report. These documents define the minimum codes for conducting research with human beings, as well the ethical principles of beneficence, respect, and justice, which form the basis for all human research endeavors (National Commission for the Protection of Human Subjects of Biomedical and Behavioral Research [National Commission], 1979). The concept of beneficence assures that the study is structured in such a way that it will benefit—and not harm—the subjects. Researchers must then address the risks and benefits inherent in the research for all participants. Respect for persons and their right to choose to participate or not, as well as their right to cease participation at any point, is addressed through the informed consent process. Justice addresses the potential for all persons to be included in the study; no single person or group—and particularly not a vulnerable person or group—can be singled out to receive benefits or harm from the research (National Commission, 1979).

What is a human subject? Human subjects are living participants who are working with one or more researchers who are studying a phenomenon to acquire data by involvement (can be via distance; not required to be face-to-face) or data that can be used to distinguish one phenomenon from another.

## The History of the Human Subjects Protection System

**Human subject protection** began with the *Nuremberg Code*, which was developed for the Nuremberg Military Tribunal as a standard against which to judge the human experimentation conducted by the Nazis during World War II. The Nuremberg Code captures many of what are now taken to be the basic principles governing the ethical conduct of research involving human subjects. Its first provision states that "the voluntary consent of the human subject is absolutely essential." Freely given consent to participate in research is the cornerstone of ethical experimentation involving human subjects. The Nuremberg Code also provides the details implied by such a requirement—namely, capacity to consent, freedom from coercion, and comprehension of the risks and benefits involved. Other provisions require that risk and harm be minimized, that the risk/benefit ratio be determined and shared with the potential subjects of the research, that qualified investigators use appropriate research designs, and that subjects have the freedom to withdraw at any time.

Similar recommendations were made by the World Medical Association in its *Declaration of Helsinki: Recommendations Guiding Medical Doctors in Biomedical Research Involving Human Subjects*, first adopted by the 18th World Medical Assembly in Helsinki, Finland, in 1964, and subsequently revised by the 29th World Medical Assembly, Tokyo, Japan, 1975, and by the 41st World Medical Assembly, Hong Kong, 1989 (World Medical Association, 2008). The Declaration of Helsinki further distinguishes therapeutic from nontherapeutic research (Steneck, 2007).

In the United States, regulations protecting human subjects first became effective on May 30, 1974. These regulations were promulgated by the Department of Health, Education and Welfare (DHEW) and raised to regulatory status in 1966 as the National Institute of Health's (NIH) Policies for the Protection of Human Subjects. The regulations established the IRB as one mechanism through which human subjects could be protected.

In July 1974, the National Commission for the Protection of Human Subjects of Biomedical and Behavioral Research was established. The Commission met from 1974 to 1978 and issued reports identifying the basic ethical principles that should underlie the conduct of biomedical and behavioral research involving human subjects and recommending guidelines to ensure that research is conducted in accordance with those principles. Its report setting forth the basic ethical principles that should underlie the conduct of biomedical and behavioral research involving human subjects is titled *The Belmont Report: Ethical Principles and Guidelines for the Protection of Human Subjects of Research.* The Belmont Report, which is named after the Belmont Conference Center at the Smithsonian Institution, sets forth the basic ethical principles underlying the acceptable conduct of research involving human subjects. Those principles— respect for persons, beneficence, and justice—are now accepted as the three quintessential requirements for the ethical conduct of research involving human subjects and are discussed below (National Commission, 1979).

- *Respect for persons* involves a researcher and his or her team recognizing the personal dignity and autonomy of individuals, and providing for special protection of those persons with diminished autonomy.
- *Beneficence* entails an obligation to protect persons from harm by maximizing anticipated benefits and minimizing possible risks of harm.
- *Justice* requires that the benefits and burdens of research be distributed fairly.

The Belmont Report also describes how these principles apply to the conduct of research. Specifically, the principle of respect for persons underlies the need to obtain informed consent; the principle of beneficence underlies the need to engage in a risk/benefit analysis and to minimize risks; and the principle of justice requires that subjects be fairly selected. As was mandated by the congressional charge to the National Commission, the Belmont Report also provides a distinction between "practice" and "research." The text of the Belmont Report is thus divided into two sections: (1) boundaries between practice and research, and (2) basic ethical principles (DHHS, 2010a).

The DHHS regulations are codified at Title 45 Part 46 of the Code of Federal Regulations and became final on January 16, 1981; these regulations were revised effective March 4, 1983, and June 18, 1991. The 1991 revision involved the adoption of the Federal Policy for the Protection of Human Subjects. The Federal Policy ( "Common Rule") was promulgated by the 16 federal agencies that conduct, support, or otherwise regulate human-subjects research; the Food and Drug Administration (FDA) also adopted certain provisions. The Federal Policy is designed to make the human-subjects protection system uniform in all relevant federal agencies and departments. Additional protections for various vulnerable populations have been adopted by DHHS reflecting vulnerable populations such as pregnant women (August 8, 1975; revised January 11, 1978, and November 3, 1978), prisoners (November 16, 1978), and children (March 8, 1983, and revised June 18, 1991) (DHHS, 2010a).

An account of the history of human-subjects research and the human-subjects protection system in the United States can be found in Rothman's *Strangers at the Bedside: A History of How Law and Bioethics Transformed Medical Decision Making* and in Maloney's *Protection of Human Research*

*Subjects.* Rothman details the abuses to which human subjects were exposed, culminating in Beecher's 1966 article, "Ethics and Clinical Research," published in the *New England Journal of Medicine*, and ultimately contributing to the impetus for the first NIH and FDA regulations (Fain, 2009).

## Definition of Research

Research is a "diligent and systematic inquiry or investigation into a subject in order to discover or revise facts, theories, applications . . . " (Dictionary.com, n.d.). The intent to publish findings is generally considered as contributing to generalizable knowledge. An investigation, then, must meet certain criteria to be classified as research. Research studies are designed in an organized, logical process that can support a range of goals, from basic scientific inquiry to a qualitative research study of a specified group. Research processes, measurement, assessment, and data collection are required elements of the study itself. Essentially, research is completed in a manner that will allow findings, experiences, or understandings gleaned from the work to be generalized to the broader population. Some research involves rodents, larger animals, or even primates. These studies are evaluated differently than research involving human subjects. When humans are involved, the research processes and procedures that include consent forms and the issue of informed consent must be evaluated by an IRB (DHHS, 2010b).

The research project is usually described in a formal protocol that sets forth an objective and a set of procedures designed to reach that objective. The Belmont Report recognizes that "experimental" procedures do not necessarily constitute research, and that research and practice may occur simultaneously. It suggests that the safety and effectiveness of such "experimental" procedures should be investigated early, and that institutional oversight mechanisms, such as medical practice committees, can ensure that this need is met by requiring that "major innovation[s] be incorporated into a formal research project."

## Boundaries Between Practice and Research

Why discuss IRB when quality improvement processes and quality assessments are the foci for most clinical nurse leaders (CNLs), nurse executives, doctor of nursing practice (DNP) candidates, and other clinical doctorate students? If the IRB is predominantly focused on the ethical conduct of research, then why should quality improvement projects be reviewed by the IRB? After all, quality improvement is not research, is it? While recognizing that the distinction between research and therapy is often blurred, practice is described as interventions that are designed solely to enhance the well-being of an individual patient or client and that have a reasonable expectation of success. The purpose of medical or behavioral practice, then, is to provide diagnosis, preventive treatment, or therapy to particular individuals.

Ultimately, patients are the focus of quality improvement/process improvement projects, and their rights must be protected (Speers, 2008); the IRB process offers that protection. Similarly, community needs assessments can impact individuals and populations; thus, their protection is also warranted.

Quality improvement activities are widely regarded as critical to the effort to reduce healthcare errors and improve patient outcomes. Most can be readily distinguished from research; however, some cannot (Speers, 2008). The issue for students in nurse executive, clinical nurse leader, and DNP programs is that they are not generating new knowledge; instead, they are testing and offering translation of research findings into practice and the care of patients. To share with colleagues a project's success in improving quality of care, results are published, which brings quality improvement projects into the realm of research.

In 2007, national attention was brought to the impact of quality improvement studies on patient care. In turn, many healthcare professionals became involved in heated arguments about the differences between research and quality improvement. For example, a major care provider implemented a checklist for insertion of large intravenous lines in patients. As a part of this checklist, providers were reminded to wash their hands prior to the procedure and to wear sterile gloves and a gown. Within 3 months, IV line infection rates fell precipitously, resulting in a simultaneous reduction in costs for the provider. However, because the checklist was determined to be an intervention that impacted patients and no consent had been obtained from those patients, the Office of Human Research Protection closed down the program. This was done despite the benign nature of the intervention and the significantly positive outcomes realized for patients.

As a result of these events, more attention is now being paid to process and quality improvement projects and drives the review of projects by IRBs. The problem that most students and project managers face with regard to completion of the application to the IRB for projects is that the application uses research language, not quality improvement language. Students frequently attempt, in error, to reconcile quality improvement projects with research language, such as describing an experimental design when presenting an intervention.

The information that IRB members need with regard to quality improvement projects is generally confined to the "W" questions and answers: What will be done? Who will do it, and who will be involved in it? When will it be done (include stages)? Where will it be done, and how will it impact processes in the location(s)? Why is it necessary (include the potential impact on practice and improving health care)? In addition to these questions, the researcher/project manager needs to answer the "How" questions: How will the project unfold? How long will it take? How will the impact be measured? Clarity is essential in the application process; students and faculty should seek help on an as-needed basis.

## Applying the Ethical Principles to Both Research and Quality Improvement

The responsible conduct of research (RCR) requires investigators involved in any level of the research to complete basic training in the protection of human subjects. Scholarship in the health sciences requires a clear understanding of the ethics involved in conducting research. This basic training can be obtained through the National Institutes of Health or the Collaborative Institutional Training Initiative (CITI) modules (CITI, 2011; NIH, 2011).

### Respect for Persons

RCR training addresses the ethical principles of respect for persons. Informed consent to participate in research or a quality improvement project is required by the ethical principle of "respect for persons." It includes three elements: information, comprehension, and voluntariness.

First, potential subjects must be given sufficient information to be able to decide whether to participate, including the research procedures, their purposes, risks and anticipated benefits, alternative procedures (where therapy is involved), and a statement offering the subject the opportunity to ask questions and to withdraw at any time from the research. Incomplete disclosure is justified only if it is clear that (1) the goals of the research cannot be accomplished if full disclosure is made, (2) the undisclosed risks are minimal, and (3) when appropriate, subjects will be debriefed and provided with the research results.

Second, subjects must be able to comprehend the information that is given to them. The presentation of information must be adapted to the subject's capacity to understand it; researchers may be required to test potential subjects to assure they understand. Where persons with limited ability to comprehend are involved, they should be given the opportunity to choose whether to participate (to the extent they are able to do so), and their objections should not be overridden. Each such class of persons should be considered on its own terms (e.g., minors, persons with impaired mental capacities, the terminally ill, and the comatose).

Third, consent to participate must be voluntarily given. The conditions under which an agreement to participate is made must be free from coercion and undue influence. IRBs are especially sensitive to these factors when particularly vulnerable subjects are involved.

## Beneficence

The principle of beneficence addresses risk/benefit assessments and includes information on the probability and potential magnitude of possible harms and benefits. Researchers must define the nature and scope of the risks and benefits, while systematically assessing them. All possible harms—not just physical or psychological pain or injury—should be considered. The principle of beneficence requires both protecting individual subjects against risk of harm and considering not only the benefits for the individual, but also the societal benefits that might be gained from the research.

## *Justice*

The principle of justice mandates that the process used to select research subjects must be fair and must result in fair selection outcomes. The "justness" of subject selection relates both to the subject as an individual and to the subject as a member of social, racial, sexual, or ethnic groups.

With respect to their status as individuals, subjects should not be selected either because the researcher favors them or because they are held in disdain (involving "undesirable" persons in risky research). Further, "social justice" indicates an "order of preference in the selection of classes of subjects (adults before children) and that some classes of potential subjects (the institutionalized mentally infirm or prisoners) may be involved as research subjects, if at all, only on certain conditions" (DHHS, 1993).

# Informed Consent

The process of assuring that the participants in research or quality improvement projects are aware of their rights and the three primary principles of respect for persons, beneficence, and justice is termed *informed consent*. Informed consent documents must present the information clearly and in readily understandable language without esoteric terms or convoluted sentence structure or word use.

The two primary elements to be addressed in the informed consent process are the provision of complete information about the study/project and the understanding of the participant regarding that information. Providing information alone is not sufficient to meet the standard of informed consent—the participant must also fully understand what he or she is agreeing to as a part of the study/project.

Some key elements of informed consent were discussed previously in relation to respect for persons, beneficence, and justice. However, some populations may be fully informed and voice understanding, yet not truly understand. Such may be the case with individuals with low literacy, for example. Options for assisting those with low literacy skills include reading the consent form for the participant and allowing sufficient time for the participant time to consult with another individual, such as a family member or clergy.

Another special case arises with children who participate in research/ projects. Parents must provide consent for all minors participating in research. The children, too, must give permission (assent) to be involved in the study. In cases where higher risks are associated, the researcher may be required to obtain assent from the child and well as consent from both parents.

Typically, informed consent takes the form of a written, signed document. However, waiver of written informed consent can be approved if the presence of a signed document could increase the risk associated with participation. The waiver applies only to the written signed document; it does not apply for the actual process of informing the participants.

## Institutional Review Board Processes and Procedures

Having to complete an IRB application can appear to be quite complicated and off-putting, but the process actually is straightforward and procedurally oriented. When one considers that the overall purpose of the IRB is to protect human subjects, the process becomes fairly benign.

IRB reviewers look for clear explanations of what will be done, who will do it, when it will be done, and how it will be done, so that the board members can determine if the project requires full board review or is eligible for expedited or exempt status. A clear understanding of the intent of the project is critical to the IRB review process. The discussion that follows highlights some ways to respond to the nature of the question without categorizing the quality improvement project in research terms while assuring ready understanding by IRB review teams. Some of the areas of the application are readily discernable, and others take a bit more information.

The remainder of this section provides details on the information needed to complete an IRB application. The basic processes the application will follow during the staged review are also addressed.

### Research Purpose

Typically, the researcher needs to provide a brief description of the intent of the project. This section is basically the same for research studies or quality improvement projects. The applicant needs to answer the question, What is the problem and which impacts will the proposed research/project have?

## Subject or Population

Who will be involved in the project and how? To which population will the results be generalizable? Again, this section is the same for research studies or for quality improvement projects. Basically, the information presented must allow investigators, institutions, or IRBs to determine if the proposed methods of selecting participants could result in unjust distributions of the burdens and benefits of research. For example, subjects should not be selected simply because they are readily available in settings where research is conducted, or because they are "easy to manipulate as a result of their illness or socioeconomic condition" (DHHS, 1993).

## Design of the Study

This section is very different for research studies and quality improvement projects. The applicant will need to provide enough information for reviewers to determine if the design fits the purpose and has the potential to yield the anticipated outcomes.

For research studies, the discussion of study design should address the overall nature of the study—experimental, quasi-experimental, descriptive, or something. Applicants must provide specific aims that the research will address and explain how the design will facilitate achieving those aims.

For quality improvement (QI) studies, the QI design, like the research design, must be linked to the project and to the project site. Some typical QI designs are the FADE model (focus, analyze, develop, and execute), PDSA (plan, do, study, act), and Six Sigma. Six Sigma actually encompasses two different models: DMAIC (define, measure, analyze, improve, control) and DMADV (define, measure, analyze, design, verify), which are used for existing and new processes, respectively. The basic premise is the same no matter which design is specified: Reviewers must know how the project will be conducted.

## Privacy and Confidentiality

How will the researcher protect the information collected? Will participants be recognizable? Will responses be linked to participants? How and where will the data be stored? Who will have access? This last issue is particularly relevant to staff or patient participants who may fear retribution if they answer questions truthfully. In QI projects, participant pools are typically smaller and site-specific. The researcher must carefully assure that the privacy of all participants is protected.

## Inclusion/Exclusion Criteria

How will the researcher determine eligibility of participants? The applicant must describe the processes and procedures used in determining who is eligible to participate in the research/project versus who is not eligible. The researcher will also need to assure that the issue of vulnerability is addressed. Frequently, quality improvement projects do not include children or other vulnerable populations, although that is not a hard-and-fast rule. Consequently, the researcher must describe inclusion and exclusion criteria comprehensively. If a population or subgroup is excluded for any reason, the application must clearly address those criteria. The researcher must be aware that the IRB application may require a stipulation whether or not any vulnerable population is included.

## Risks and Benefits from Participation

Even if they are minimal, the researcher needs to address all risks and benefits to the participant, actual or potential, including physical and psychological risks and benefits, inconvenience, and loss of privacy. If subjects will be paid to participate in the research, the amount of payment and the restrictions on the payment need to be explained in detail. With regard to risks and benefits, more attention is generally paid to the risks than to the benefits. Therefore, the IRB members must independently assess the risk to the participants to determine if they agree with the risk assessment in the application. Additionally, the IRB must determine the type, probability, and extent of the risk as much as possible. It must determine if the researcher's estimates of harm or benefit to participants are reasonable, given the facts and results of other studies.

Five basic principles apply to risk/benefit assessment:

1. "Brutal or inhumane treatment of human subjects is never morally justified."
2. Risks should be minimized, including the avoidance of using human subjects if at all possible.
3. IRBs must be scrupulous in insisting on sufficient justification for research involving "significant risk of serious impairment" (direct benefit to the subject or "manifest voluntariness of the participation").
4. The appropriateness of involving vulnerable populations must be demonstrated.
5. The proposed informed consent process must thoroughly and completely disclose relevant risks and benefits (IRBNet, 2012).

## Outcomes

The researcher must describe how the findings will be used. Are the findings sufficient to propose a change in policy or practice, or will more research be needed with different groups, under different circumstances, or some other criterion?

For QI projects, will the project potentially change practice? How might that change occur? Who will the change affect?

## Informed Consent Form

A copy of the informed consent document is included in the packet provided to the IRB so that an assessment can be made with regard to the accuracy of information shared with participants and the reading level required to assure true understanding.

# Levels of Institutional Review Board Reviews

The IRB has the authority to approve or not approve research and/or QI projects (Fain, 2009). IRB reviews occur on three distinct levels depending on the degree to which the study is considered to constitute potential harm or violation of one or more ethical principles. Those three levels are full review, expedited, and exempt (Polit & Beck, 2012). An applicant can request a specific level of review, but the final decision regarding that level rests with the IRB staff and committee.

The full review process requires that a full IRB committee, including scientific, nonscientific, and community members, evaluate the study. All members of the IRB read, consider, and evaluate each study. Primary and secondary reviewers are stipulated to present the salient facts of the study to the full board, including all components of human-subject protection. The researcher maintains responsibility for the responsible conduct of research, even with a full board review. A full board review is typically reserved for studies with inherent risks to participants. Examples of studies that fit this criterion are those focused on sensitive topics such as race, ethnicity, and sexual behaviors; studies focused on vulnerable populations; and clinical trials, especially related to medication regimens.

Expedited reviews are reserved for studies in which "minimal" exposure to risk is projected. Minimal risk is defined as the participant being at no greater risk than he or she could encounter as a part of daily life. Expedited reviews are typically, conducted by one or two members of the IRB committee and are reported at the IRB meeting but not discussed there. Many QI projects qualify for an expedited review, as they constitute minimal risk to subjects.

An exempt review designation is typically reserved for studies where no human subjects are involved or for studies where there is no risk to humans. Typically, exempt studies include situations where subjects cannot be identified, secondary review of existing data, studies in which data are gathered through observation of public behavior, and anonymous surveys (DHHS, 2010a).

## Summary

- This chapter has provided an overview of the role of the institutional review board (IRB) in an organization, a review of the basic processes involved in the review of a study, and methods involved in the protection of human subjects.
- The institutional review board is the primary mechanism used by institutions to assure the protection of human subjects through informed

consent, justice, beneficience, and respect for persons. The institutional review board also reviews quality improvement studies to assure that human subjects are protected.

- Researchers must be aware of the institutional review board policies within their institutions and be prepared to complete the processes to assure the protection of the persons involved in their research.

## Reflection Questions

1. Which institutional criteria are used to review an IRB application?
2. What differentiates a quality improvement project from research?

## References

Collaborative Institutional Training Initiative (CITI). (2011). CITI course in the responsible conduct of research. https://www.citiprogram.org/rcrpage.asp?language=english&affiliation=100

Dictionary.com. (n.d.). "Research" definition. Retrieved from http://www.dictionary.reference.com/browse/research?s=t

Fain, J. A. (2009). *Reading, understanding, and applying nursing research* (3rd ed.). Philadelphia, PA: F. A. Davis.

IRBNet. (2012). Innovative solutions for compliance and research management. https://www.irbnet.org

National Commission for the Protection of Human Subjects of Biomedical and Behavioral Research. (1979). The Belmont report: Ethical principles and guidelines for the protection of human subjects of research. http://www.fda.gov/ohrms/dockets/ac/05/briefing/2005-4178b_09_02_Belmont%20Report.pdf

National Institutes of Health (NIH), Office of Extramural Research. (2011). Protecting human research participants. http://phrp.nihtraining.cm/users/login.php

Polit, D. F., & Beck, C. T. (2012). *Nursing research: Generating and assessing evidence for nursing practice* (9th ed.). Philadelphia, PA: Lippincott Williams & Wilkins.

Speers, M. A. (2008). Editorial: Quality Improvement: Research or non-research? AAHRPP perspective. *Association for the Accreditation of Human Research Protection Programs, Advance, 5*(2), 1–2.

Steneck, N. H. (2007). *ORI: Introduction to responsible conduct of research.* U.S. Department of Health and Human Services. http://www.ori.hhs.gov/publications/ori_intro_text.shtml

U.S. Department of Health and Human Services (DHHS). (1993). Institutional Review Board Guidebook. http://www.hhs.gov/ohrp/archive/irb/irb_introduction.htm

U.S. Department of Health and Human Services (DHHS). (2010a). Code of federal regulations. http://www.hhs.gov/ohrp/humansubjects/guidance/45cfr46.html#46.html#46.102

U.S. Department of Health and Human Services (DHHS). (2010b). Guidance on IRB continuing review of research. http://www.hhs.gov/ohrp/policy/continuingreview2010.html

U.S. Department of Health and Human Services (DHHS). (2011). Information related to advanced notice of proposed rulemaking (ANPRM) for revisions to the Common Rule. http://www.hhs.gov/ohrp/humansubjects/anprm2011.page.html

U.S. Department of Health & Human Services (DHHS). (2012). The federal policy for human subject protections (The Common Rule). http://www.hhs.gov/ohrp/humansubjects/commonrule/index.html

World Medical Association. (2008). World Medical Association Declaration of Helsinki: Ethical principles for medical research involving human subjects. http://www.wma.net/en/30publications/10policies/b3/index.html

# Case Exemplar

## ■ CASE STUDY 1

### The Role of Research in Policy Development

*Jennifer Styron and Ronald A. Styron, Jr.*

Two researchers were interested collecting data regarding the types of cyberbullying collegiate students experienced in high school (grades 9–12), the effects of cyberbullying, and those who tend to serve as cyberbullies. The project was two-pronged. Part I of this research project was intended to provide school administrators and educators with information that they would find useful when developing policies and practices surrounding the safe use of technology and peer bullying. Part II sought to collect data to determine the level of cyberbullying students experienced on campus, the means by which students dealt with such cyberbullying issues, and the level of student awareness regarding campus resources.

## Reflection Questions

1. Based on the research proposed, would this study be best suited for exempt, expedited, or full IRB review?
2. Are there foreseeable risks to conducting the study? If so, does this violate the principle of beneficence?
3. Is there a risk of privacy/confidentiality breaches in the proposed research?

## ■ CASE STUDY 2

### Evaluating Interprofessional Education

*Sheila Whitworth and Jennifer Styron*

The aim of this study was to explore key themes found through a year-long interprofessional clinical experience. Emerging themes from the program's evaluation were expected to provide insights into the development of leadership and competency skills of nurses, physician assistants, and medical students. Findings were to be utilized to make program improvements and provide insight into effective teaching and learning strategies specific to leadership and communication competency development in interprofessional clinical settings. Solicited students would include only the students who attended an interprofessional experience over the course of the project period (August 2013 through July 2014). This group included students from the physician assistant, medical, and nursing programs. Informed consent processes were followed, but no signed consent was obtained. The primary investigator provided each participant with a copy of the consent agreement. Voluntarily participating in the project implied participant consent.

## Reflection Questions

1.  Do studies that primarily focus on program evaluation need to go through the IRB process? Why or why not?
2.  Is it acceptable to provide informed consent but not require a signature prior to participation in the study? Does this still adequately address respect for persons, beneficence, and justice?
3.  Was the population solicited representative for the aims of the study?

# ■ CASE STUDY 3

## Accelerated Nursing Program and Faculty Efficacy

*Sheila Whitworth and Jennifer Styron*

The purpose of this project was to identify best practices of accelerated nursing programs and the characteristics of faculty teaching in accelerated programs. This project addressed three research questions: (1) the efficacy of curricular design of accelerated programs; (2) the characteristics of faculty teaching in accelerated nursing programs and the differences, if any, in teaching methods when compared with those who teach in hybrid or traditional programs; and (3) best practices for the recruitment of future faculty. Findings from this study provided insight into accelerated program development and curriculum that will further address the national issue of healthcare professional shortages and the need for highly educated nurses and nursing faculty.

Using a mixed-method design, project leads developed two quantitative instruments and conducted a regional pilot study to accelerated prelicensure programs that were institution members of the Southern Regional Education Board (SREB). This allowed the project team to understand programmatic models, faculty attributes, and resources and support needed for accelerated faculty. In total, 62 institution members with accelerated prelicensure programs, including 40 institution members with baccalaureate programs and 22 institution members with master's accelerated programs, were available for participation. In addition, solicitation for participation included faculty from the selected sample teaching in traditional or hybrid programs.

## Reflection Questions

1. Would this proposal be considered research or quality improvement?
2. Were the inclusion/exclusion criteria utilized for this proposed research appropriate?
3. Did the proposed outcomes substantiate the need for this study?

# ■ CASE STUDY 4

## The CNL Capstone Project: An Experiential and Transformative Process

*Theodora Ledford*

Differentiating quality projects from research often challenges students to ensure that the objective of the project is met and any impact on human subjects' protection is determined. Upon completing a microsystem needs assessment and engaging in dialogue with the institutional review board, it was established that the clinical nurse leader (CNL) project was needed to obtain information that supported nursing quality improvement data. Data gleaned from the project would be useful for detecting trends in and patterns of performance that affected more than the identified microsystem. Data collected would be utilized in the development of action plans in collaboration with other practice committees concerning nurse-sensitive indicators directed at quality, safe, and efficient patient outcomes. Additionally, data could engender interprofessional collaboration, opportunities to monitor and evaluate compliance with standards, recommendations to enhance continuous quality improvements, and the spread of safety initiatives throughout the healthcare system.

While the capstone project started initially as an outcomes-based endeavor where differentiating quality improvement from research was of foremost importance, the transformative processes that followed were valuable. The experience culminated in thoughts of how unit-based quality nursing councils could use data to create more solid structures and processes. As a result, an innovative environment was envisioned where strong professional practice would flourish and the mission, vision, and values would come to life. This notion can become a reality. However, during dialogue with colleagues and quality improvement staff, a fundamental action was needed—namely, the development of a guide for other nurses to understand the differences between quality improvement projects and research and the steps necessary for accomplishing meaningful and value-added quality projects that are patient-centric and advance care delivery. Steps are in process for the action to become reality.

# Reflection Questions

1. Which individual challenges do students confront when completing IRB applications for universities and clinical agencies?
2. How might students create opportunities from challenges associated with quality improvement and research endeavors?

## CHAPTER FOUR

# Synergistic Interprofessional Teams: Essential Drivers of Patient-Centered Care

*Patricia L. Thomas*

## *Chapter Objectives*

1. Describe tools, strategies, and methods used to create synergistic interprofessional teams that are dedicated to effective project planning, management, and patient-centered programs.
2. Discuss the importance of synergy, change theory, transformational leaders, creativity, and innovation as interprofessional teams construct process tools applicable to practice.
3. Assess the value and use of various metrics when evaluating interprofessional team effectiveness and measurable outcomes.

## *Key Terms*

| | | |
|---|---|---|
| Ad hoc team | Leader | SBAR communication |
| Brainstorming | Multidisciplinary team | Synergy |
| Collaboration | Program management | Task force |
| Interdisciplinary team | Project planning | Team |

## *Roles*

| | | |
|---|---|---|
| Leader | Manager | Team member |

## *Professional Values*

| | | |
|---|---|---|
| Evidence-based practice | Integrity | Quality |

## *Core Competencies*

| | | |
|---|---|---|
| Appreciative inquiry | Design | Leadership |
| Assessment | Interpersonal | Management |
| Critical thinking | relationships | Project management |

# Introduction

Much has been written about the importance of interprofessional learning, the development of interprofessional teams, and the contributions and roles nurses will be expected to make and fill, respectively, as new care-delivery systems and practice settings evolve. Several distinct models have been developed to showcase the changes needed in practice and academe, yet implementation of these models and resultant sustained outcomes have been slow, sporadic, and inconsistent. Principles and constructs for teamwork, team building, and facilitating teams are extensive, spanning decades of work in nursing, business, and social sciences. Recent alignment of these concepts with safety, quality, and high reliability has catapulted the structure and process of teams and investment in team skills to the forefront. In this chapter, aligning principles of project management with the larger landscape of interprofessional teams is the focal point. Emphasis is placed on "how to do this" rather than "why we do this," given the general agreement that project work can be accomplished only through productive, high-functioning teams.

Recent landmark reports from the Institute of Medicine (IOM) and the Robert Wood Johnson Foundation have highlighted that while healthcare practitioners claim to value teamwork, communication, **collaboration**, and shared outcomes, we are plagued by professional assumptions, definitions, habitual use of language, and power structures. Notably, in the IOM's *To Err Is Human* report (1999), preventable errors were attributed to organizational structures, incomplete information, failures in communication, and faulty systems and pro cesses rather than to people. Likewise, the IOM's *Crossing the Quality Chasm* report (2001) emphasized that healthcare systems are not always able to translate knowledge into practice related to quality and safety in large part because resources are not used effectively in fragmented systems where gaps and redundancies create waste and fail to achieve desired outcomes. The six aims to improve patient care—that is, making such care safe, effective, patient-centered, timely, efficient, and equitable—are cornerstones to project management given expectations for cost-effective, high-quality care found in mission, vision, and value statements throughout the healthcare industry. Implied in this focus is the realization that, despite our best efforts, we have not accomplished these aims consistently and as an industry. Transformative change and investments in organizational capacity, information infrastructure-building, and retraining of multidisciplinary care teams are needed (IOM, 2001). The Robert Wood Johnson Foundation and Institute of Medicine's *Future of Nursing: Leading Change, Advancing Health* report (2010) made further recommendations about how to transform the nursing workforce through education, leadership development and competencies, and use of data and information to address the gaps apparent in the current delivery systems.

In light of these reports and recommendations, alignment and understanding of team dynamics, synergies that can be generated, and the need for creative and innovative models implemented by nurse led teams are needed. Basic to this work is an appreciation for what exists today, which voids and gaps are present, and how new strategies and competencies must be leveraged.

## Fundamentals of Teams

Concentrating on **project planning** and **program management**, determination of when the efforts of an individual versus the efforts of a group or team are needed is pivotal to success. Sometimes, individual choices, decisions, or actions enable success. Indeed, historically, the belief was held that individual actions, decisions, and accountability alone brought results. Based on this perspective, silos of information and action were created, only to produce inconsistent and fragmented results, ineffective communication, and poor outcomes. We have since learned that success coming from collective efforts in complex systems rests in the ability to draw distinctions between when individual effort (commitment, participation, and actions) versus facilitated team efforts bring greater efficiency, effectiveness, and consistency aimed toward desired results. As part of the latter approach, the role of the project manager becomes more systematic, guiding group or team members to shared goals, shared language, and **synergy**.

### *Teams Versus Groups*

The distinction between teams and groups is a foundational concept, yet one that is often overlooked. Groups and teams hold attributes in common, but differentiation between their attributes can sometimes explain why projects or programs become derailed. Groups and teams hold in common the gathering of individuals who will work together to accomplish goals. What distinguishes groups from teams is how extensive the interdependence of members is, how they are led, and who has ownership for the end product of the members' interactions. Group members have individual accountability to complete work; come together to share information; complete individual work or tasks based on their role; are focused on their own challenges and interests; and have a purpose and goals that are directed by a manager. In contrast, team members have individual and mutual accountability; come together for discussion, problem solving, and planning; focus on collective goals and work products; and have a purpose, work, and goals that are shaped by the **leader** in conjunction with the members (Brounstein, 2002).

Analogies are often offered using sports examples to showcase the differences between groups and teams. With this being the case, marathon runners would an example of a group. These athletes have gathered for the same purpose, want to win, and share common interests. By comparison, in baseball, soccer, or football teams, individual players come together but have to rely on one another to win. They have common goals but depend on the direction of the coach and the decisions and actions of their team members to ultimately achieve victory. An individual could have a "great game" yet still lose. For the purposes of project and program management, building teams rather than groups is the desired state.

We all hold unspoken assumptions that the goals and desired outcomes of people within the same organization are the same, simply because we care for the same patients and work with a common mission and vision statement to guide our work. We might recognize differences between disciplines, roles, or levels of authority, but spend little time in setting of expectations or confirming definitions in the language we use to ascertain interdependence. Additionally, we may use words and believe we hold common definitions, only to find that our education and experiences have shaped our underlying assumptions in ways that are not consistent with how others view the same situation. This diversity underlies the miscommunication challenges that can lead to harm.

Another important distinction in health care is that between a **multidisciplinary team** and an **interdisciplinary team**. Although these terms are often used interchangeably, they have very different meanings. The healthcare literature, depending on the discipline or specialty, uses these terms to signal levels of accountability. Interdisciplinary teams recognize the interdependence of members who come together to understand complex situations or solve complex problems that require the knowledge, skills, and abilities of diverse individuals who cannot be successful without one another. In this coming together of the individuals, recognition of overlapping roles is common, and unraveling the distinctions between them leads to an understanding of how the various members' contributions could be woven together in a unique way to bring a new or different result. In contrast, multidisciplinary teams engage the knowledge, skills, and abilities of the members who work in parallel with distinct responsibilities to accomplish a shared goal. Interdisciplinary teams bring out synergy and new possibilities, whereas multidisciplinary teams reinforce consistency in defined disciplinary outcomes (Nancarrow, Booth, Ariss, Smith, Enderby, & Roots, 2013; Walters, 2012).

## Team Structures

As with clarifying language about **teams**, it is important to understand how words are used to describe the structure of teams and the duration of work they have been charged to accomplish. Committees, **task forces**, **ad hoc teams**, and councils represent common structures (and language) in healthcare organizations. Their permanency, charter, and purpose often determine how and why a team is established and guide the relevance attributed to organizational work. Committees and councils may result from expectations held by regulators (like The Joint Commission or state regulations) or governing boards and have defined responsibility and authority directed toward ongoing work. In contrast, task forces and ad hoc teams are often created to address an issue or need that has arisen. As such, their work is typically geared toward making recommendations aimed at an issue with the intent of informing leaders and then disbanding (or transitioning into a newly created committee or council) (Danna, 2013; Walters, 2012).

Danna (2013) identified six rules of synergy and team building that are pivotal to interprofessional team effectiveness:

1. *Define a clear purpose.* Each team member must clearly be knowledgeable about the reason the team is coming together. Team members must also be able to articulate the goals, objectives, and purpose of the team.

2. *Actively listen.* Each team member must be focused on each individual and listen to what is being said. Active listening is not judgmental and means being completely absorbed and attentive to the speaker.

3. *Maintain honesty.* Each team member must be objective in providing feedback to the speaker. No one should make the speaker feel belittled or suggest that his or her view is not correct or important.

4. *Demonstrate compassion.* Each team member should listen in a caring manner to the others' viewpoints.

5. *Commit to resolution of conflicts.* Each team member must agree to disagree when his or her view or opinion is not the same as the other members'. Team members must work toward a common understanding and acceptance of the issue at hand.

6. *Be flexible.* Each team member must be open and flexible to other individuals' perspectives. Everyone must work together to accomplish the goal or objective.

## Developmental Stages for Teams

Irrespective of the team's purpose, composition, or expected duration, certain phases or stages of development can be anticipated and observed in teams. The interactive behaviors exhibited between members during these phases reflect the dynamic interplay between individual and group behaviors that support the identity of the team. A commonly cited model for the developmental team phases comes from the work of Bruce Tuckman (1965). His model is helpful in understanding the normalcy of group dynamics, moving from coming together, to finding cohesiveness and synergy, to producing outcomes, and finally to dissolving:

- *Forming:* During this orientation phase, members define interpersonal boundaries and task behaviors.
- *Storming:* Members resist group influence or task requirements, such that this phase is characterized by interpersonal conflict.
- *Norming:* Resistance declines and cohesion emerges as expectations and roles are accepted. Members feel free to share thoughts and ideas.

- *Performing:* Members are productive and work for the common goal of the group. Interpersonal relations drive activities and results (Tuckman, 1965).
- *Adjourning:* The team dissolves because the tasks have been completed and the goals achieved (Tuckman & Jensen, 1977).

During the forming phase, the team members discover themselves and want to preserve their uniqueness or individuality. The goals and tasks for the team are offered, and individuals establish why they may have been selected for the team and how they can contribute to its work. The focus is on individual interests, and testing comes in the form of establishing acceptable behaviors. The exchange of information is high as the group establishes ground rules and members size one another up. As the group is formed, selecting content experts and persons who have implemented solutions is common. Attention to different problem-solving styles and ensuring equal numbers of sensing/thinking versus intuitive/feeling members is key. This will benefit the group in the performing stage (but may be a source of conflict expressed in the storming phase). The group leader develops the explicit norm of constructive conflict by addressing disagreement, multiple definitions, minority opinions, the role of the "devil's advocate," and a "group wins" psychology (Antai-Otong, 2013; Danna, 2013; Walters, 2012).

In the storming phase, members of the group jockey for position, control, and influence. Competition becomes apparent and leadership struggles ensue. The honeymoon phase of orientation has ended, and work requirements become evident. Resistance to the group influence emerges, and intragroup conflict may arise. During this stage, team members have low levels of trust and often display anger and resentment. While turf battles may ensue, the foundations for trust and respect may be developed during this stage based on how conflicts are resolved. The leader supports the team by assisting with assignments and group roles, conflict resolution, and enforcement of the ground rules that were developed in the forming phase (Antai-Otong, 2013; Danna, 2013; Walters, 2012).

In the norming phase, cohesion is developed as roles and norms are established to move the group toward consensus. Members share a common understanding of the opportunity to reach group goals, and there is openness to alternative definitions and multiple views. Morale and trust are high and negativity is suppressed. Open communication during this phase facilitates constructive discussions and the sharing of personal and professional insights (Antai-Otong, 2013; Danna, 2013; Walters, 2012).

In the performing phase, members work with deep involvement, greater disclosure, and unity. Because they are bound together by common goals, productivity is high and team synergy is evident as members rely on their collective talents to accomplish work. Loyalty to the team is evident and efforts revolve around quality of team product. This is the phase where work is completed and the leader is less involved (Antai-Otong, 2013; Danna, 2013; Walters, 2012).

In the adjourning phase, team tasks are completed and the outcomes of the work lead to self-evaluation by the team and its members. There can be sadness and mourning because team members have accomplished tasks and goals and will now move on (Antai-Otong, 2013; Danna, 2013; Walters, 2012).

While the process is described here as a series of sequential phases, team formation is not always linear. Phases may be repeated, interrupted, or skipped. With the entry of a new team member, the departure of a team member, new leadership, or revised goals and deliverables, the team may shift to an earlier or later phase to find equilibrium (Antai-Otong, 2013; Danna, 2013; Walters, 2012).

Having an understanding and awareness of these phases is important for the project or program manager, because they explain behaviors that may be observed at different points in team development. Given that many teams bring together individuals with diverse backgrounds (professionally) and experiences (in terms of tenure and previous work on teams), guidance during each of these phases can help teams work through the developmental milestones in an appropriate manner. For example, recognizing that conflict during certain phases actually brings harmony and productivity in subsequent stages, the project manager who understands storming as a developmental phase can preserve his or her energy and resist intervening. If conflicts arise in the performing phase, the project manager might take a different approach to intervene if the conflict persists, as one would expect the interpersonal relationships of the team members would typically address conflict and come to a resolution (Antai-Otong, 2013; Tuckman, 1965; Walters, 2012).

## Barriers to Effectiveness in Teams

While each member joins a team with a sense of hope and anticipation, there are times when barriers arise that decrease the effectiveness of teams. Common pitfalls include an inability to trust or rely on team members, fear, unresolved conflict, lack of commitment, low standards and the avoidance of accountability, and attention to personal gain rather than the results of the team. Each of these pitfalls can be avoided with effective leadership.

Initially, the program planner's or project manager's role is to assist team members in developing trusting relationships by demonstrating reliance on them to overcome limitations of knowledge, skills, or abilities that may be demonstrated by individual team members. The team leader can demonstrate vulnerability and call on the members of the team to step forward and fill the gap.

Fear and unresolved conflict require team leaders to support constructive debates and demonstrate the ability to manage these negative emotions by establishing group norms for dealing with issues in a manner that is respectful to all team members.

When a lack of commitment is evident, the underlying problem is likely a lack of decision-making capacity by the team, such that individuals seek consensus instead of taking a clear position on issues. This can be resolved through inclusion of all points of view in making decisions. Similarly, a lack of accountability can be countered by assisting the team to focus on goals, continually tracking team progress, and communicating frequently with the team through meetings and status reports.

Finally, inattention to the results of the team can be minimized through the selection of measures that clearly define success for the team effort (not individual interests) and the development of a tracking mechanism to monitor team progress. Success and failures must be equally shared within the team and used to reinforce progress to goals.

## Strategies for Work Management

The work of a team to improve processes can be both challenging and rewarding. Effective leadership is facilitated through the use of structures and tools to ensure participation by all members of the team. The use of standardized communication tools to support teamwork within the complexity of the healthcare environment has been explored in the literature as a means of improving decision making and increasing safety (O'Daniel & Rosenstein, 2008).

Deliberate and distinct strategies to improve communication, define accountability, and establish routines in health care have drawn marked attention in recent years, in large part driven by the analysis of errors and their root causes and a commitment to improve quality, safety, effectiveness, and efficiency through recommendations from the IOM (1999, 2001). Four of these strategies are highlighted here: Team STEPPS as a curriculum and framework for teams and organizations, **brainstorming** and nominal voting as strategies for teams, and **SBAR (situation, background, assessment, recommendations) communication** as a means for individuals to support effective communication between professionals and departments.

## Team STEPPS

Created by the Agency for Healthcare Research and Quality (AHRQ) and the Department of Defense, Team STEPPS is an evidence-based teamwork model that was developed to describe necessary skills and behaviors for team outcomes. The model includes skills for leadership, mutual support, situation monitoring, and communication. Feedback cycles are used with specific tools for communication, to plan, and to deliver care. Tools such as briefings, team huddles, and SBAR communication are the foundation from which fewer errors and improved outcomes flow (AHRQ, n.d.; Danna, 2013).

## Brainstorming and Nominal Group Voting

Brainstorming has become a widely embraced strategy and tool to give equal voice and weight to members of team in quality improvement work. Brainstorming sessions generate a large number of ideas coming from team members, directed toward team goals. Individuals call out ideas that are recorded on a board or flip chart in a sequenced fashion until no more ideas can be generated. The essential rules of brainstorming are that everyone participates and that no discussion, critique, or evaluation of the ideas takes place during the session. A benefit of this strategy is that it brings to light options and ideas that may not have been previously considered, as judgment is suspended and all members of the team have equal standing in the process irrespective of title, role, or tenure. Creative and innovative thoughts often emerge. Once all ideas have been recorded, subsequent discussions can focus on feasibility (Koch, 2013; Walters, 2012).

Similarly, the nominal group process starts with a stated objective and proceeds with each member writing his or her own list of possible solutions. Time is given to draft responses, with members then taking turns in sharing ideas with the group. As with brainstorming, ideas are not discussed until all have been presented. Once the list of ideas is complete, clarification follows (Koch, 2013; Walters, 2012).

Once ideas are generated using brainstorming or nominal group processes, the team proceeds to pare down the list of suggestions by such mechanisms as voting to eliminate ideas that are not feasible, identifying items that may be readily implemented (low-hanging fruit), and rank-ordering related alternatives. Having individual team members rank each idea and then calculating average scores for each idea to determine the degree of agreement among team members can accomplish rank ordering. Clarification and discussion of the strengths, weaknesses, opportunities, and threats (SWOT) of each idea can be undertaken by the team as well. Additionally, an affinity diagram, in which ideas are written on cards and placed randomly on a table or chart, can be generated. Like or related ideas are then placed together by group members working silently. When cards are no longer being moved, the group discusses the ideas and generates a title for each group. Each of these methods can prove useful in exploring alternative plans of action toward goal attainment.

## SBAR Communication

When communication patterns between physicians and nurses were examined by researchers, a common experience was that nurses felt unprepared. Developed by Kaiser Permanente and recommended by the Institute for Healthcare Improvement, the SBAR technique aims to improve communication by establishing a structure that supports critical thinking, setting expectations for consistency in informational elements. The SBAR template includes the situation (concern, problem, or issue), background (the clinical context, assessment (what the individual has ascertained about the situation), and recommendations (the corrective action needed).

First, the situation is outlined by providing a brief summary of what is going on. This is followed by background information about the clinical situation or the context of the issue. The assessment component presents a statement of what the individual has identified as the problem and is followed by a recommendation of which corrective action is needed. Originally developed to facilitate communication between nurses and physicians, the use of the standardized SBAR format as part of team communication dynamics provides a succinct method of communicating information rapidly. Given the successes achieved with the use of this tool, SBAR has become a standardized method for team and interdepartmental communication in many organizations (Malloch & Porter-O'Grady, 2010; Walters, 2012).

## Synergy and Creativity

While the essence of project or program management is a systematic and disciplined approach to leading people through change and the completion of tasks, it also provides the opportunity to bring new ideas, relationships, and enthusiasm to an organization. The confidence of the team leader in navigating pitfalls and bringing people deliberately through the achievement of milestones is expected. What may be overlooked is the opportunity for creativity and transformation—outcomes that are often realized by teams led by seasoned project managers. In times of great change or uncertainty, it is easy to draw from past experiences and conform to rules or practices that brought success in the past. Appreciative inquiry, coupled with project management skills and quality improvement structures, can move teams from transactional interactions to transformational results and warrants attention given the expectations placed on us during the era of health reform.

While difficult to define, synergy is a product of effective work teams. Such an experience is commonly cited by as one of the benefits and satisfiers realized when working in a highly effective team. As individuals become members of a team and successfully work through the developmental stages, their energy, respect, and anticipation of positive outcomes buoy the members as they recognize the products and outcomes of coming together. Additionally, the enthusiasm and spirit of possibility are shared with individuals outside the work team while sharing experiences and implementing change.

Although it is not equivalent to professional development and team identity, the synergy experienced by members of teams is often described as growth derived from the relationships, feedback, and insights gained from the experience. Attributes that contribute to the synergy emerge through the interactions of team members supported by active listening, contributing, motivation, and cognition (Malloch & Porter-O'Grady, 2010). This group-level phenomenon has been described as an unconscious process of the group that manifests in individual group member actions, thereby creating positive or negative outcomes collectively that are very different from the outcomes that would have been achieved by simply adding up the contributions of the individuals. Part of the synergy comes from active listening and openness of team members as they explore options that might have been dismissed by an individual, lending to the collective creativity. Another part of the synergy comes from the self-correcting function of teams, as they counteract undesired outcomes and position the team to capitalize on individual and group creative assets.

## Appreciative Inquiry

While often thought of as a strategic lever for leadership and change, appreciative inquiry (AI) has applications relevant to project and program management in light of the need to preserve clinical outcomes and quality metrics, while simultaneously modifying those things that have been unresponsive to change initiatives. At its core, appreciative inquiry is the art and practice of asking questions that strengthen a system's capacity to apprehend, anticipate, and heighten positive potential. By focusing on what *is* working rather than what is not, AI shifts thinking away from the typical "what is not working" perspective and guides us to greater acknowledgment and preservation of those things that are functioning as desired. Rather than finding deficits and gaps, AI brings attention to strengths within teams or organizations and highlights those things that can be replicated.

Cooperrider's (1990) seminal work in AI describes this process as having four stages: discovery, dream, design, and destiny. Discovery is the mobilization of the team or system into a positive change core. The dream stage occurs when a transparent, results-oriented vision is created through discovering potential and asking questions that identify a higher purpose. Design occurs when possibilities are realized regarding the ideal state and people feel capable of expanding the positive core by developing new dreams and concepts. Destiny evolves from the strengthening of the positive capabilities and capacities of the system, building hope and momentum focused on deeper purpose. Because members of the organization feel safe and energized, a space for learning, adjustment, and improvisation is created (Thomas & Roussel, 2013).

By mobilizing a spirit of inquiry, AI heightens the group's collective imagination and innovation capabilities rather than focusing on what is not working in a project, program, or organization. The language of AI is different from the current state, given that critical analysis and identification of what is not working take more time and attention than the celebration of what is working.

Hubbard (1998) views AI as a conscious evolution of realities in the new century. This process recognizes social construction by focusing on metaphor, ways of knowing, and language, thereby producing a generative theory and advancement in action research. AI has been used in organizational development practice, as part of strategic planning, and as a framework to move from problem-based management to transformational leadership and human development (Thomas & Roussel, 2013).

## Transformational Leadership

Given the need for engagement, honesty, innovation, trust, creativity, and recognition of things valued by members of teams, AI as a framework to generate solutions merits consideration. Underlying the success of AI are strong leaders with clarity, vision, and the ability to influence the thinking of others—in other words, transformational leaders. Transformational leadership has been recognized as a style of leadership that extends beyond transactions. It includes the change or transformation of both the leader and the follower that occurs when leaders broaden, extend, and elevate the interests of employees, generate awareness and acceptance of the purposes and mission of the group, and stir employees to look beyond their own self-interest for the good of the group (Bennis & Nanus, 1985; Roussel & Ratcliffe, 2013). In this way, leaders serve as agents of change who influence and inspire others and then are also changed themselves.

Transformational leaders motivate followers to perform beyond normal expectations by reshaping their thoughts and attitudes and by enlisting vital support of the vision while striving for its fulfillment. This is accomplished through attributed charisma, or modeling behaviors that gain admiration and trust; inspirational motivation, or the ability to envision and articulate a future; intellectual stimulation, involving questioning assumptions and reframing problems from a new perspective; and individualized consideration, through delegation and empowerment while attending to individual needs, abilities, and aspirations (Avolio & Bass, 2002; Bass, 1990; Tomey, 2010). The theory of transformational leadership implies that people need a sense of mission that extends beyond transactions and interpersonal relationships. This is especially true in health care, where the speed of and demand for change often exceed our perceived capacity.

For project and program managers, transformational leadership offers a framework that aligns with the roles and expectations many will hold for their work. Empowerment of others, clarity in vision, and expectations of transformative change through the leadership of teams generate synergy and creative possibilities not previously considered. Through the ability to influence others, build trust, and support teams as they press through their work to accomplish goals, transformative leadership brings extraordinary results. Aspiring to become a transformational leader is within the reach of project and program managers.

# Innovation

Much has been published on the need to hardwire evidence-based practices into the healthcare environment. Recently, attention has shifted from evidence to innovation. Porter-O'Grady and Malloch (2015) pointedly stated, "Innovation is not merely a process. It is a dynamic. Innovation gives new meaning and direction and challenges the historic, the expected, and the routine. It calls for innovators to adopt an attitude that reflects that all work processes and activities are subject to the discipline of constant inquiry and reassessment" (p. 155).

The challenge for the interprofessional team is not how to generate new ideas and opportunities, but rather how to make innovation a deeply entrenched aptitude and competency in any project endeavor (Gibson, 2014). The innovative project team should ensure that the integrity and sustainability of the project's outcomes can adapt to the changing demands of both the internal and external environments, and that the collective interest of the organization is advanced by those outcomes. Producing value in a singular innovative project can create opportunities for additional value-based opportunistic projects. Sustained project outcomes and effective teams are the goal of and standard for high-functioning innovative systems, where a culture of innovation is valued and respected. Missed opportunities occur daily in clinical settings and life in general. Harnessing the energy and talents of an interprofessional team will turned missed opportunities into an innovation pipeline that produces high-quality, safe, and effective outcomes that benefit varying populations and communities.

## Summary

- Effective project and program management depends on the ability to facilitate teams and guide them to successful goal attainment.
- Time spent on understanding team dynamics is time well spent, but should be followed by leadership development to support and sustain trust, satisfaction, and accomplishment of goals by creating a space where curiosity and innovation are the norm.
- The five stages of team development—forming, storming, norming, performing, and adjourning—are the platform on which effective teams can be built.

- The challenge to synergistic, interprofessional teams is to adopt an aptitude of innovation that is disciplined, constantly inquiring, and reassessing.
- Strategies directed toward building trust, effective communication, curiosity, and innovation will serve organizations well as they address the demands placed on the industry for healthcare delivery redesign.

## Reflection Questions

1.  You are assigned to lead a project to reduce readmissions to your hospital. The chief executive officer (CEO) has identified the first priority as preventing unnecessary readmissions from skilled nursing facilities and home care agencies that your health system owns. Who would you request to be on this team and why? What would be your first steps?

2.  You have been asked to step in and chair a subcommittee of the Quality and Safety Committee of the board of directors. This subcommittee has been charged with creating a patient safety program, and the leader of this group has been on a leave for three months. The trends by unit show increasing falls with injury and increasing medication errors despite barcode scanning. After reviewing the team charter and the outcomes dashboard for the work of this subcommittee, you realize the team has stalled, and the metrics and measures of success have not changed for more than a year despite the subcommittee's practice of meeting monthly. You know you will need to make some changes to achieve the team charge. You have been asked to write your plan for a meeting with the CEO and the chief nursing officer (CNO) tomorrow. What would you include in your plan? Which recommendations might you make regarding selection of new team members? Will you recommend disbanding this team and starting with new members? To manage expectations, what would you emphasize to the senior executives in terms of the team composition, timing, and future meetings?

3.  You have been asked to join a newly created organizational team tasked with creating the strategy and processes to increase department-specific innovations to fulfill the Triple Aim. After you listened to the team's

discussion, you walked away feeling like the team did not have a clear definition of what innovation is. You decide to call the team chair to meet for lunch so you can learn how "innovation" will be defined. Based on what you know about the discipline and rigor involved in project and team leadership, who else in the organization would you want to talk to before the next meeting? Which approach might you take with the team to generate ideas? Which resources would you tap to assess the organization's past successes with change and innovation?

# References

Agency for Healthcare Research and Quality (AHQR). (n.d.). Team STEPPS national implementation. http://teamstepps.ahrq.gov/about-2cl_3.htm

Agency for Healthcare Research and Quality (AHQR). (n.d.). Team STEPPS: Strategies and tools to enhance performance and patient safety. http://www.ahrq.gov/professionals/education/curriculum-tools/teamstepps/index.html

Antai-Otong, D. (2013). Effective communication and team collaboration. In J. L. Harris, L. Roussel, & P. Thomas, *Initiating and sustaining the clinical nurse leader role: A practical guide* (2nd ed., pp 105–140). Burlington, MA: Jones & Bartlett Learning.

Avolio, B., & Bass, B. (2002). *Developing potential across a full range of leadership: Cases on transactional and transformational leadership.* Mahwah, NJ: Lawrence Erlbaum Associates.

Bass, B. (1990). *Bass and Stogdill's handbook of leadership: Theory, research, and managerial applications* (3rd ed.). New York: NY: Free Press.

Bennis, W., & Nanus, B. (1985). *Leadership: The strategies for taking charge.* New York, NY: Harper & Row.

Brounstein, M. (2002). *Managing teams for dummies.* New York, NY: Wiley.

Cooperrider, D. (1990). Positive image, positive action: The affirmative basis of organization. In S. Srivastva & D. L. Cooperrider (Eds.), *Appreciative management and leadership* (pp. 91–125). San Francisco, CA: Jossey-Bass.

Danna, D. (2013). Organizational structure and analysis. In Linda Roussel, *Management and leadership for nurse administrators* (6th ed., pp 213–307). Burlington, MA: Jones & Bartlett Learning.

Gibson, R. (2014). The no. 1 challenge to innovation. http://www.innovationexcellence.com/blog/2014/09/14/the-no-1-challenge-to-innovation/

Hubbard, B. (1998). *Conscious evolution: Awakening the power of our social potential.* Novato, CA: New World Library.

Institute of Medicine (IOM). (1999). *To err is human: Building a safer health system.* Washington, DC: National Academies Press.

Institute of Medicine (IOM), Committee on Quality of Health Care in America. (2001). *Crossing the quality chasm: A new health system for the 21st century.* Washington, DC: National Academy Press.

Koch, M. (2013). Quality management: Key to patient safety. In Linda Roussel, *Management and leadership for nurse administrators* (pp 619–645). Burlington, MA: Jones & Bartlett Learning.

Malloch, K., & Porter-O'Grady, T. (2010). *Introduction to evidence-based practice in nursing and health care* (2nd ed.). Sudbury, MA: Jones and Bartlett.

Nancarrow, S., Booth, A., Ariss, S., Smith, T., Enderby, P., & Roots, A. (2013). Ten principles of good interdisciplinary team work. *Human Resources for Health.* http://www.human-resources-health.com/content/11/1/19, doi: 10.1186/1478-4491-11-19

O'Daniel, M., & Rosenstein, A. (2008). Professional Communication and Team Collaboration in Patient Safety and Quality: An Evidence-Based Handbook for Nurses, http://www.ncbi.nlm.nih.gov/books/NBK2637/

Porter-O'Grady, T., & Malloch, K. (2015). *Quantum leadership: Building better partnerships for sustainable health* (4th ed.). Burlington, MA: Jones & Bartlett Learning.

Robert Wood Johnson Foundation & Institute of Medicine (IOM). (2010). The future of nursing: Leading change, advancing health. http://www.thefutureofnursing.org/sites/default/files/Future%20of%20Nursing%20Report_0.pdf

Roussel, L., & Ratcliffe, C. (2013). Transformational leadership and evidence-based management in a changing world. In L. Roussel, *Management and leadership for nurse administrators* (6th ed., pp 729–756). Burlington, MA: Jones & Bartlett Learning.

Thomas, P., & Roussel, L. (2013). Clinical nurse leadership: Creating the vision. In J. L. Harris, L. Roussel, & P. Thomas, *Initiating and sustaining the clinical nurse leader role: A practical guide* (2nd ed.). Burlington, MA: Jones & Bartlett Learning.

Tomey, A. (2010). *Guide to nursing management and leadership* (8th ed.). Terre Haute, IN: Mosby-Elsevier.

Tuckman, B. (1965). Developmental sequence in small groups. *Psychological Bulletin, 63,* 384–399.

Tuckman, B., & Jensen, M. (1977). Stages of small group development revisited. *Groups and Organizational Studies, 2,* 419–427.

Walters, S. (2012). Team power and synergy: Project planning and program management essentials. In J. L. Harris, L. Roussel, S. Walters, & C. Dearman (Eds.), *Project planning and management: A guide for CNLs, DNPs, and nurse executives* (pp 39–50). Burlington, MA: Jones & Bartlett Learning.

# Case Exemplar

## ■ CASE STUDY 1

### Emotional Intelligence: A Catalyst for Interprofessional Team Success

*Margaret Mitchell*

All behavior has a purpose and consequences, whether they are recognized at the moment of action or at a later time during self-reflection. Failure to recognize how one reacts to situations and subsequent interactions with others can be a deterrent to individual and team success. Interactions among team members drive outcomes and successful change. If a member of a team is resistant or reactive during a situation and is unaware of this behavior, the entire team may suffer. A project's potential outcomes may therefore be unattainable or significantly reduced. The interactions, relationships, and emotional intelligence of team members are, in turn, vital to individual (evolutionary) or team (revolutionary) change in today's chaotic healthcare environment. If these are overlooked, opportunities for team synergy and mindfulness are reduced, if not lost. Being mindful of recurring situations, past reactions, and emotions can only improve the odds for interprofessional team synergy and success.

Numerous authors have recognized the importance of emotional intelligence as a determinant for achieving personal and team excellence (Bradberry & Graves, 2009; George, 2000; Goleman, 1998). According to Goleman (1998), emotional intelligence determines the potential for learning the practical skills of emotional competence. Appreciation and governance of one's emotions and those of the team can help alleviate team conflict as team activities and interprofessional projects evolve (George, 2000). Bradberry and Graves (2009) and Goleman (1998) advocate reinvestment in beliefs and values as a means to redirect disruptive impulses that are prone to suspend judgment and to help the individual think before acting. Failing to handle or even consider one's actions or consider the feelings of others limits team synergy and any sustainable outcomes. This may further diminish the commitment and motivation of any team both in the immediate term and in the long-range future (Porter-O'Grady & Malloch, 2015).

Throughout their careers, nurses and other professionals are required to interact with one another. Observing how individuals respond to members of their own discipline, especially nurses, can be particularly enlightening, as the phrase "We eat our own" is commonplace when listening to nurses in conversation. Being mindful of how an experienced nurse responds to a new graduate nurse can be directly attributed to the former's emotional intelligence and can directly impact this relationship. A negative response or action can create conflict, and when individuals are unaware of their own negativity or reactivity in such a situation, this behavior may in turn be observed in interactions with others.

While there are no guarantees that these lessons will change how one reacts to any situation or crisis, thought leaders have offered several insights into means of enhancing emotional intelligence and potentially bringing about effective and sustainable interprofessional team synergy (Goleman, 1998; Porter-O'Grady & Malloch, 2015):

- Openness to novel ideas
- Valuing the knowledge and expertise of others
- Compassion
- Resilience
- Passion toward accomplishing a team goal
- Impulse control

The value attached to emotional intelligence can be exploited to advance a team's function and outcomes. Team members who are attuned to self and use their emotional intelligence wisely can be beneficial to outcomes and sustained success. Being open to serendipitous and developing influences that occur expectedly is a hallmark of both an emotionally intelligent team member and an effective team. Such influences can improve care delivery and advance health care in the 21st century and beyond.

## Reflection Questions

1. How might emotional intelligence affect the outcome of a team of which you are a member?
2. Which of your personal strengths and attributes advance team functioning? How are these attributes used in your daily practice environment?

## References

Bradberry, T., & Graves, J. (2009). *Emotional intelligence 2.0*. San Diego, CA: TalentSmart.

George, J. (2000). Emotions and leadership: The role of emotional intelligence. *Human Relations, 53*(8), 1027–1055.

Goleman, D. (1998). *Working with emotional intelligence*. New York, NY: Bantam.

Porter-O'Grady, T., & Malloch, K. (2015). *Quantum leadership: Building better partnerships for sustainable health* (4th ed.). Burlington, MA: Jones & Bartlett Learning.

## CHAPTER FIVE

# Managing the Interprofessional Project Team

*James L. Harris and Kathryn M. Ward-Presson*

## *Chapter Objectives*

1. Recognize the key elements of managing interprofessional teams during projects in a competitive and chaotic healthcare environment.
2. Explore the importance of a common language shared by clinical and administrative project planners and managers.
3. Translate the characteristics of coaching interprofessional teams in the planning, initiating, and evaluating phases of projects.
4. Describe the needs of interprofessional teams and the significance of team leadership in maintaining continuous performance given the mandates imposed by accrediting agencies and stakeholders.

## *Key Terms*

| | | |
|---|---|---|
| Collaboration | Interprofessional team | Performance |
| Communication | Language | Team synergy |
| Interdisciplinary team | Organizational culture | |

## *Roles*

| | |
|---|---|
| Coach | Leader |

## *Professional Values*

Quality

## *Core Competencies*

| | | |
|---|---|---|
| Assessment | Emotional intelligence | Leadership |
| Communication | Evaluating | Management |
| Coordination | Innovation | Policy management |
| Design | Interpersonal | |
| Diversity | relationships | |

# Introduction

Health care remains at a crossroads, as patients' medical conditions become increasingly more complex, reimbursement and regulatory mandates expand and intensify, and knowledge emerges from a series of catalyzing changes that challenge care delivery globally. As innovative quality projects are planned and applied, engagement of **interprofessional team** members and their continuous management are vital to success. Speaking a common **language** and understanding the meaning of each term and concept translates into significant outcomes and **team synergy**. Knowledge gleaned from projects requires mobilization of the evidence through continuous **communication** and consciousness-raising if innovation is to be sustained (Crisp, 2014). When various disciplines engage in interprofessional projects, education, and collaborative practice, high-quality, safe, and efficient care is realized (Interprofessional Education Collaborative [IPEC] Expert Panel, 2011; World Health Organization [WHO], 2013).

This chapter discusses the essentials in managing interprofessional teams that are engaged in clinical and quality projects, and emphasizes the importance of using a common language in all phases of projects, their management, and collaborative efforts. The value of coaching interprofessional project teams is also addressed as a means to capitalize on team **performance** given the changing healthcare landscape being driven by new and existing accrediting, regulatory, and stakeholder demands.

## Interprofessional Teams: Overview and Management

Achieving optimal outcomes is a hallmark of any team effort. However, sustaining those outcomes requires ongoing engagement, commitment, collaborative interprofessional practice, and management. The concepts of interprofessional teams and collaborative practice are not foreign ideas to healthcare professionals. Zaccagnini and White (2014), for example, support the notion that effective interprofessional teamwork and **collaboration** include not just vested professionals, but other stakeholders and team members from various disciplines. A well-orchestrated and -assembled project team may require the inclusion of patients as well as professionals from technology, health policy management, and library science. Rigorously aligning and integrating the needs and interests of individuals collectively creates a transformative connection. Ideas can be generated, shared, and communicated toward a defined aim. This approach can guide projects, add value, and create avenues for managing processes and conflicts that may arise during any project team effort. Value, whether directly or indirectly, indicates growth or improvement occurring within the team, system, or project (Dunevitz, 1997).

To provide a context for the remainder of this chapter and throughout the text, it is important to distinguish between interprofessional teams and **interdisciplinary teams** given that both terms are used—sometimes interchangeably—in the literature. These terms actually have quite different meanings. Zaccagnini and White (2014) distinguish "interprofessional" as signaling the inclusion of representatives from a particular discipline or knowledge branch with differing experiences, education, values, roles, and expectations. By comparison, "interdisciplinary" is more specific to a particular discipline. Generally, "interprofessional" is associated with a broader definition and context as related to projects, collaborative efforts, and their management.

The rapidity of change in the healthcare industry has necessitated support of understanding and integrating management and leadership, as interprofessional project teams have proved able to generate novel approaches for meeting the increasing demands made by consumers and the healthcare industry itself. Managing a successful team that is dedicated to improvement and practice change requires the development of reciprocal trust and continuous interpersonal relationships among team members (Kouzes & Pozner, 2007). If time is not allowed for teams to progress through developmental stages, managing the team will be almost impossible, and the potential gains from a team's synergy will be lost. In 1965, Tuckman proposed a model for group stages that has proved valuable in understanding a team's development. A final stage was later identified that further supported team synergy (Tuckman, 2001). These five stages—forming, storming, norming, performing, and adjourning—are discussed next.

*Forming* is the initial stage in which the team comes together for the purpose of completing a defined project aim. During this stage, trust is essential as the team members get to know one another, form interpersonal relationships, clearly articulate the group's aim, and further define their roles and responsibilities.

In the *storming* stage, team trust has not fully developed and conflicts may arise due to differing disciplines, opinions, and lived experiences. Communication and directly approaching conflicts are essential actions by the team leader at this stage. The complexity of individual differences, gender, culture, ethnicity, language, and emotions can limit communication, however, such that further conflicts may ensue. Conflicts are frequent when there is resistance to change. Some individuals may be satisfied with the status quo and threatened by change; they require the leader to openly address this stance lest opportunities to meet a goal or aim and learn from others are diminished. Unresolved conflict reduces productivity, lowers team morale, and is costly (Chinn, 2008; Feldman, 2008; Patterson, Grenny, McMillian, & Switzler, 2002).

The emotional intelligence of team members and the team leader is of upmost importance during the storming stage. Emotions can become a barrier to moving forward as a productive team to accomplish the specific aim (McCallin & Bamford, 2007). Emotional intelligence (EI) is a valuable leadership attribute in terms of the awareness of the role played by emotion in communication, rapport building, and motivation. According to Goleman (1998), EI determines the potential for learning the practical skills of emotional competence and is divided into five realms:

- Self-awareness: The ability to recognize and understand one's emotions, moods, and drives, as well as the effects on others.
- Self-regulation: The ability to handle emotions so they do not interfere with project work yet to be completed.
- Motivation: The desire to engage in work beyond personal reasons
- Empathy: The ability to understand the emotions of others.
- Social skill: Skill in relationship management and network building needed to meet a common understanding and rapport.

As an attribute of the leader, EI is credited with contributing to many successes and often plays a more significant role than cognitive abilities as the project team progresses in its work (Goleman, Boyzatsis, & McKee, 2002).

*Norming* is the next stage, where team identity begins to develop. During this stage, open dialogue is promoted in which ideas and differing insights are shared and accepted. The team leader needs to be alert to preventing groupthink at this point, as it could inhibit progression to the next stage.

As the *performing* stage matures, team loyalty and assets of team members are used to full benefit. Territorial differences by professionals need to be removed, as flexibility is a common indicator of the ability to accomplish the project's stated aim. Finally, in the *adjourning* stage, performance and progress are evaluated in terms of the outcomes.

Throughout each of these stages, a shared purpose, trust, respect and recognition, collaboration, shared responsibility, and mutual decision making are markers for successful progression. Healthcare systems are complex, adaptive systems requiring flexibility, collaboration, use of a common language by team members, and responsibility for the ultimate project aim to be met and patient-centered care accomplished (Begun, Zimmerman, & Dooley, 2003).

## A Common Language: A Driver for Interprofessional Project Team Success

Interprofessional project teams are composed of individuals from varying backgrounds, both clinically and culturally. Developing and adopting a mutually agreed-upon common language can only benefit the project and functions as a driver for team success and measurable outcomes for future replication.

Central to the team leader's role is understanding the communication preferences of various generations represented on the project team. In a technology-driven environment, the challenge of making rapid changes and responding to identified issues may hinder a project team unless the communication preferences of various generations are considered and used to benefit the project aim (Martin & Tulgan, 2006). **Table 5-1** describes some of the communication preferences by generation. Keeping these pointers in mind when leading and managing project teams will prove beneficial to a positive product.

Unintentional and various jargon used by project team members can also hinder the progress of the team. It is not uncommon to observe different disciplines or individuals with personal agendas from a specific discipline who have priorities that compete with the project aim. For example, on a pain management project team, different disciplines or individuals may differ in terms of their preferred pain assessment techniques, observations, and descriptors; in

**Table 5-1**  Communication Preferences by Generation

| Generation | Spoken Preference | Written Preference |
|---|---|---|
| Traditionalists (Birth years: 1900–1945) | Formal linear thinkers, direct and to the point, no foul or offensive language, no small talk, proper grammar. | Well organized, proper grammar and punctuation, to the point, like written communication for future reference. |
| Baby Boomers (Birth years: 1946–1964) | Like small talk to build consensus and foster teamwork. | Written word for later reference and creation of paper trail preferred. |
| Generation X (Birth years: 1965–1980) | Informal and direct with little to no small talk. Focus is on what things mean for them. | Little preference for reading; desire concise bullet points with outcomes clearly delineated. Little focus on grammar and punctuation. |
| Millennials (Birth years: 1981–2000) | Prefer spoken communication if the message is very important; desire others to show respect through language spoken; prefer action verbs with important messages; desire use of language to portray visual pictures; not skilled at personal communication because of the technical ways of communicating used during their lifespan. | Use positive, respectful, motivational electronic communication style; portray pictures through language; use action verbs. May need direction on written communication formats. |

turn, these differences may create a barrier to accomplishing the aim of developing a mutually agreeable language and process for documenting and describing a patient's pain experience.

As noted previously, communication barriers are created when others do not comprehend the language, which then limits opportunities for mutual idea and knowledge sharing. Kaiser Permanente developed the standardized tool known as SBAR (situation, background, assessment, and recommendation) communication to deal with this risk. Interprofessional teams use the SBAR tool for discussion and solving patient problem situations; it provides a succinct method for ensuring team information exchange in a rapid cycle. Project teams also find this tool useful for achievement of project milestones (Leonard, Graham, & Bonacum, 2004).

Project teams may also benefit from other shared, common language as projects are envisioned and implemented. For example, the National Patient Safety Goals and the Institute of Medicine's (IOM) Six Safety Aims highlight contributions by interprofessional teams in achieving desired, measurable collaborative goals (IOM, 2001; National Patient Safety Goals, 2014). Many projects today focus on quality, safety, efficiency, and opportunities in an effort to demonstrate sustainable outcomes with replicable measurement and generation of empirical data. Language included in Lean, Six Sigma, and other methodologies offers a sustainable means of engaging in projects that emphasize the continuum of care, care coordination, pay for performance, and at-risk contracting for payment (Naylor, 2012).

An organization's culture plays an important role in how information is communicated and language is used, and both of these factors influence every project plan and activity. **Organizational culture** also plays an important role in all healthcare processes and the interchanges between patients and providers. Organizations that engender ingenuity of project improvements teams and remove an entrenched "culture of blame" in favor of a "just culture" will prevail in these turbulent times. Notably, safer practices will follow when the just culture approach is adopted (Scott-Cawiezell, Jones, Moore, & Vojir, 2004). Just cultures foster supportive environments in which staff can questions practices, express concerns, and admit mistakes without punishment (Tucker, Nembhard, & Edmondson, 2007).

If an organization is able to promote interprofessional project teams that invest their efforts in advancing practice and creating empirical evidence, it is likely to have fewer incidents and system failures than an organization that holds on to the traditional "culture of blame" (Khatri, Brown, & Hicks, 2009). Incorporating the language of just culture and being true to its meaning will continuously foster positive team function and sustainability. Hence, high-reliability organizations are realized in which care is safe and errors are minimized while achieving exceptional performance in quality, safety, and efficacy (LaPorte, 2006).

## Coaching Interprofessional Project Teams

Teams are the driving force to success in any organization. Whether they form a functional team, a team of managers, or a specific project team, people collaboratively working together produce effective outcomes. As part of interprofessional team socialization, coaches assist members throughout all phases of a project. Coaches act as connectors who know lots of people. Their importance extends beyond the *number* of people they know to the *kinds* of people they know (Gladwell, 2002). A coach uses this information when working with teams to assist them in recognizing the value of all members and the importance of demonstrating interprofessional respect toward one another. Otherwise, the performance and productivity of a project suffer.

Hanson and Spross (2009) posit that a paradox of the current healthcare system is the existence of both incentives and disincentives for interprofessional team members and organizations to collaborate. Both the incentives and the disincentives play powerful roles, such that motivation to collaborate is eliminated by a counterforce. Recognizing this paradox will assist interprofessional project teams in seizing opportunities for strategic and sustainable collaboration in supportive environments.

Team coaching can be a powerful tool as teams work together to accomplish a specific aim. Coaching is a method used for support, encouragement, and career development (Finkelman & Kenner, 2010). Equally important is showing teams how to reduce conflict and improve working relationships for achievement of an identified aim.

Coaching a team requires this leader to focus on skills and interactions versus individual development. Interactions with team members and their

communication are central to effective performance. One of the initial characteristics of a successful coach is understanding the team dynamics and translating this information throughout the phases of the project so as to attain the
desired outcomes. Identifying how team members relate to one another is important for decision making and productivity. Indeed, member behavioral assessments often prove beneficial for improving a team's productivity. As a coach,
encouraging group discussion of behavioral assessments assists members to see
one another differently, understand other people's perspectives, and adapt individual behavior for improved results. To realize this outcome, the team coach
must ensure that a clear set of behavior expectations is mutually established and
maintained to eliminate individual preferences that might otherwise obscure the
project aim. Defining processes for team members to follow will support this
endeavor.

Recognizing the need to evaluate reward and recognition systems and support individual development are the final roles of a team coach. When team
members have personal goals that do not match with the goals of the team, problems may potentially arise. In such a case, the coach needs to identify sources of
competing values and ensure that reward systems align correctly with individual
performance. Being supportive of individual development is important for the
coach as well, as members ideally will gain insights and attain new skills that
ultimately benefit them individually in future team activities as well as the current project (Edmonson, 1999; Hall & Weaver, 2001).

In summary, Hackman and Wageman (2005, p. 283) suggest that team
coaching will foster effectiveness only when four conditions are present:

1.  The group performance processes that are key to performance effective-
    ness (i.e., effort, strategy, and knowledge and skill) are relatively uncon-
    strained by task or organizational requirements.
2.  The team is well designed and the organizational context within which it
    operates supports rather than impedes teamwork.
3.  Coaching behaviors focus on salient task performance processes rather
    than members' interpersonal relationships or on processes that are not
    under the team's control.

4.  Coaching interventions are made at times when the team is ready for them and able to deal with them—that is, at the beginning for effort-related (motivational) interventions, near the midpoint for strategy-related (consultative) interventions, and at the end of a task cycle for (educational) interventions that address knowledge and skills.

## Leading Interprofessional Project Teams Based on Needs and Mandates

Despite widespread agreement in disciplines about the centrality of clinical experiences to knowledge acquisition, extensive findings about the teaching practices or learning opportunities that foster interprofessional healthcare teams' outcomes remain limited. Such knowledge will benefit acquisition of the knowledge and skills needed to design and implement interprofessional projects resulting in safe, quality care. The extent to which individuals are best positioned to lead effective clinical or administrative project teams reflects needs, competencies, and competing mandates.

The 21st-century technologies, accreditation standards, and stakeholder demands for teamwork, communication, and coordination rely heavily on evidence to inform processes and care delivery. Identifying the needs of interprofessional project teams highlights the importance of leading them to engage in continuous improvement. Likewise, leaders and teams who possess interprofessional competencies and understand the interrelationships between patients and the team will facilitate project completion and satisfaction of the mandates that often drive management actions and decisions (IPEC Expert Panel, 2011).

Leaders at all levels are challenged to shape new clinical environments and create a culture that incorporates change. This change will be influenced, managed, and ultimately evaluated as it spreads to other environments. The call to create environments and core competencies sensitive to interprofessional team needs, strengths, and cultural diversity recognizes this reality. But one may ask, why now, and which core competencies should be adopted and utilized?

The Interprofessional Education Collaborative (IPEC) Practice Competencies panel is one group that has accepted the call to action and attempted to answer this question. This panel suggested the following steps as a response:

1.  Create efforts across professions to ensure content is included in curricula.
2.  Guide curricular development toward outcomes.
3.  Provide foundations for a learning continuum across professions that embrace and engender lifelong learning.
4.  Acknowledge that evaluation and empirical inquiry strengthen scholarship related to interprofessional competencies.
5.  Prompt dialogue to identify goodness of fit between core competencies, practice, needs, and mandates (IPEC Expert Panel, 2011, p. 7).

In addition, the IPEC panel identified four domains of interprofessional collaborative practice (**Table 5-2**) and desired principles of the interprofessional competencies (**Box 5-1**).

While the competency domains and specific competencies are general in nature and function, there is mutual agreement that they can position leaders of interprofessional teams to be successful. As teams accomplish project aims, mandates posed internally and externally will be met. However, project leaders must ensure that the team is aware of the realities inherent in any change and recognize that adaption is even more important than anticipation (Porter-O'Grady & Malloch, 2015).

Managing any team, whether a clinical project team or a systems change team, requires leaders to keep in mind that the membership of the interprofessional team is a partnership among professionals, individuals, families, and

**Table 5-2** Interprofessional Collaborative Practice Domains

Competency Domain 1: Values and Ethics for Interprofessional Practice

Competency Domain 2: Roles and Responsibilities

Competency Domain 3: Interprofessional Collaboration

Competency Domain 4: Teams and Teamwork

*Source:* IPEC Expert Panel, 2011, p. 16.

---

| **Box 5-1** | Desired Principles of Interprofessional Competencies |
|---|---|

- Patient centered
- Community and population oriented
- Relationship focused
- Process oriented
- Developmental learning activities, strategies, and behavioral assessments specific to the learner
- Integration across the continuum of learning
- Sensitive to systems and the applicability across all care settings
- Applicable across professions
- Stated in common and meaningful language across professions
- Outcome driven

*Source:* Republished with permission of Association of American Medical Colleges, from Core Competencies for Interprofessional Collaborative Practice, James L. Harris and Kathryn Ward-Presson, © 2011; permission conveyed through Copyright Clearance Center, Inc.

---

communities. Team leadership and management are based on expertise and competencies that match the needs of the team. Decision making and problem solving is a shared responsibility, where information provided by patients and various disciplines is key for the success of any project endeavor (Simpson, Rabin, Schmitt, Taylor, Urban, & Ball, 2001). While there is no assurance that a leader can manage a project team with 100% effectiveness, these ideas can turn the interprofessional project team into an energetic and productive enterprise.

## Summary

- Interprofessional team engagement is pivotal to quality, safe, and effective project outcomes.
- The five stages of team synergy include forming, storming, norming, performing, and adjourning.
- Using a common language that interprofessional team members understand and endorse will advance care delivery and continuous improvement.

- Coaching project teams requires leadership competencies as well as an understanding of interprofessional core competencies, the basic assumptions of team functioning, and guiding principles for productive and positive deliverables.
- As interprofessional team needs and competencies are identified, team leaders can capitalize on them to meet the project aim and create a productive enterprise.

## Reflection Questions

1.  For a member of an interprofessional project team, which characteristics are essential for efficient and effective management of the team toward accomplishing the identified aim? How could you use the leader characteristics to lead a project team to successful outcomes?
2.  How can the use of a common language by project team members enhance or inhibit success?
3.  What are two primary needs of successful interprofessional teams? Discuss how you might use this information to meet various mandates in the current healthcare environment.

## References

Begun, J., Zimmerman, B., & Dooley, K. (2003). Health care organizations as complex adaptive systems. In S. M. Mick & M. Wyttenback (Eds.), *Advances in health care organization theory.* San Francisco, CA: Jossey-Bass.

Chinn, P. (2008). *Peace and power.* Sudbury, MA: Jones and Bartlett.

Crisp, N. (2014). Mutual learning and reverse innovation: Where next? *Crisp Globalization and Health, 10*(14), 1–4.

Dunevitz, B. (1997). Perspectives in ambulatory care: Collaboration—in a variety of ways—creates health care value. *Nursing Economics, 15*(4), 218–219.

Edmondson, A. C. (1999). Psychological safety and learning behavior in work teams. *Administrative Science Quarterly, 44,* 350–383.

Feldman, H. (2008). *Nursing leadership: A concise encyclopedia.* New York, NY: Springer.

Finkelman, A., & Kenner, C. (2010). *Professional nursing concepts: Competencies for quality leadership.* Sudbury, MA: Jones and Bartlett.

Gladwell, M. (2002). *The tipping point: How little things can make a big difference.* New York, NY: Back Bay Books/Little, Brown.

Goleman, D. (1998). *Working with emotional intelligence.* New York, NY: Bantam.

Goleman, D., Boyzatsis, R., & McKee, A. (2002). *Primal leadership: Realizing the power of emotional intelligence.* Boston, MA: Harvard Business School Press.

Hackman, J. T., & Wageman, R. (2005). A theory of team coaching. *Academy of Management Review, 30*(2), 269–287.

Hall, P., & Weaver, L. (2001). Interdisciplinary education and teamwork: A long and winding road. *Medical Education, 35,* 867–875.

Hanson, C. M., & Spross, J. A. (2009). Collaboration. In A. B. Hamric, J. A. Spross, & C. M. Hanson (Eds.), *Advanced practice nursing: An integrative approach* (4th ed.). St. Louis, MO: Saunders Elsevier, *10,* 283–314.

Interprofessional Education Collaborative (IPEC) Expert Panel. (2011). *Core competencies for interprofessional collaborative practice: Report of an expert panel.* Washington, DC: Interprofessional Education Collaborative.

Institute of Medicine (IOM). (2001). *Crossing the quality chasm: A new health system for the 21st century.* Washington, DC: National Academies Press.

Khatri, N., Brown, G. D., & Hicks, L. L. (2009). From a blame culture to a just culture in health care. *Health Care Management Review, 34*(4), 312–322.

Kouzes, J., & Pozner, B. (2007). *The leadership challenge.* San Francisco, CA: Wiley.

LaPorte, T. A. (2006). High reliability organizations: Unlikely, demanding and at risk. *Journal of Contingencies and Crisis Management, 4*(2), 60–71.

Leonard, M., Graham, S., & Bonacum, D. (2004). The human factor: The critical importance of effective teamwork and communication in providing safe care. *Quality and Safety in Health Care, 13*(suppl 1), 85–90.

Martin, C. A., & Tulgan, B. (2006). *Managing generational mix: From urgency to opportunity.* Amherst, MA: HRD Press.

McCallin, A., & Bamford, A. (2007). Interdisciplinary teamwork: Is the influence of emotional intelligence fully appreciated? *Journal of Nursing Management, 15*(4), 386–391.

National Patient Safety Goals. (2014). http://www.jointcommission.org/standards_information/npsgs.aspx

Naylor, M. (2012). Achieving high value transition care: The central role of nursing and its leadership. *Nursing Administration Quarterly, 36*(2), 115–126.

Patterson, K., Grenny, J., McMillian, R., & Switzler, A. (2002). *Crucial conversations: Tools for talking when stakes are high.* New York, NY: McGraw-Hill.

Porter-O'Grady, T., & Malloch, K. (2015). *Quantum leadership: Building better partnerships for sustainable health.* Burlington, MA: Jones & Bartlett Learning.

Scott-Cawiezell, J., Jones, K., Moore, L., & Vojir, C. (2004). Moving from a culture of blame to a just culture in the nursing home setting. *Nursing Forum, 41,* 133–140.

Simpson, G., Rabin, D., Schmitt, M., Taylor, P., Urban, S., & Ball, J. (2001). Interprofessional healthcare practice: Recommendations of the National Academies of Practice expert panel on healthcare in the 21st century. *Issues in Interdisciplinary Care, 3*(1), 5–19.

Tucker, A. L., Nembhard, I. M., & Edmondson, A. C. (2007). Implementing new practices: An empirical study of organizational learning in hospital intensive care units. *Management Science, 53,* 894–907.

Tuckman, B. W. (2001). Development sequence in small groups. *Group Facilitation: A Research and Applications Journal, 3,* 66–81.

World Health Organization (WHO). (2013). Interprofessional collaborative practice in primary health care: Nursing and midwifery perspectives: six case studies. *Human Resources for Health Observer, 13.* Geneva, Switzerland: Author.

Zaccagnini, M. E., & White, K. W. (2014). *The doctor of nursing practice essentials* (2nd ed.). Burlington, MA: Jones & Bartlett Learning.

# Case Exemplar

## ■ CASE STUDY 1

### Transforming Care with Engaged Teams

*Kathryn M. Ward-Presson*

## Background

Visionary leadership and interprofessional collaboration among all members of the healthcare leadership team is essential to improve patient care outcomes and meet Triple Aim objectives (Bisognano & Kenney, 2012). As a member of the "C Suite," the chief nursing officer (CNO) routinely works with other executives such as the chief executive officer (CEO), chief of staff (COS), chief operating officer (COO), and chief financial officer (CFO) to identify organizational goals and determine clinical outcome measures and commensurate targets requiring priority focus. Goals and outcome measures identified should be consistent with those established by the facility's board of directors. Achieving goal attainment and the sustainability of improved patient outcomes depends on the selection of healthcare leadership team members who demonstrate effective project management and collegial problem-solving competencies (American Nurses Association, 2009; American Organization of Nurse Executives, 2007; Harris, Roussel, Walters, & Dearman, 2011).

## Nursing's Role

The CNO and other nursing leaders hold pivotal roles that may positively influence the achievement of organizational quality improvement objectives. One example of that influence is seen with the successful execution of designated projects such as the implementation of clinical bundles to address patient outcome deficits. This is especially true when the organization's priority projects involve nurse-sensitive indicators such as rates of hospital-acquired pressure ulcers (HAPU) and catheter-associated urinary tract infections (CAUTI).

## Facility Exemplar

The existence of higher than target (0%) HAPU and CAUTI rates in a large tertiary teaching and research healthcare facility provides an example highlighting strategies to improve these rates through the collaborative efforts of the facility's nursing staff and other members of the team. Creating effective senior and mid-level nursing leadership teams was essential to the nursing team's ability to work collegially with other disciplines and address unit-based (microsystem) and overall nursing (macrosystem) performance improvement (PI) initiatives. Any improvements achieved due to nursing interventions and partnerships with non-nurse colleagues also served to improve the organization's HAPU and CAUTI rates at the macrosystem level.

The CNO employed a variety of leadership assessment strategies (e.g., one-on-one sessions with each senior nursing leadership member, Strengths Finder 2.0 assessments [Rath, 2007], and small group meetings) to determine senior nursing leadership team members' interests, strengths, challenges, and career goals. Each member's ability to work with all nursing staff and other disciplines was also examined. Individual professional development plans were implemented to assist with each member's growth and competency development. Similar strategies were adopted by senior nursing leaders when assessing and establishing development plans for their direct-report nurse managers.

Establishing a senior nurse leader role of "Performance Improvement and Practice" and identifying an individual to fill this position (someone who possessed the necessary advanced competencies in the application of evidence-based practice principles, data gathering, and analysis and staff engagement) was critical to providing oversight for nursing PI projects, a central repository for performance-related information, and the availability of a subject-matter expert to assist line staff with unit-based and global PI projects. The facility's existing nursing shared governance structure was also evaluated and strengthened to ensure staff participation reflective of all job categories throughout the continuum of care.

Nursing wound care specialists led the facility's wound care committee and engaged committee members from other disciplines (medicine, infection control, dietary, materials management, and pharmacy) to ensure the creation of an interprofessional forum to address needed improvements in policies, procedures, and processes related to the organization's pressure ulcer prevention program. The committee reviewed evidence-based HAPU bundles and led the rollout of the designated HAPU bundle on an organization-wide basis. This group also monitored HAPU bundle implementation progress and reported relevant outcomes data to the medical and nursing executive committees and the governing body. Similar interprofessional team creation and operational strategies were employed to address the facility's CAUTI bundle implementation and outcome monitoring/reporting project.

The facility's unit-based and overarching nursing PI committees and the Nurse Executive Council (NEC) were updated at least quarterly regarding progress toward meeting the 0% HAPU and CAUTI rate targets. Unit-based PI committees and NEC members evaluated the data, provided input regarding further opportunities to improve the efforts, and determined strategies that appeared to be more effective than others in decreasing either rate. Results and reports were presented visually in the form of graphs and run charts, and raw numbers with benchmarks were shared during small and large group meetings. Results were also posted on unit bulletin boards for all stakeholders to review. The information provided also included narrative discussions about the effectiveness of the interventions used. Summary information was incorporated in the organization's annual nursing report as well.

With the support of the organization's executive team, senior nursing leadership and the NEC developed another strategy to improve HAPU and CAUTI outcomes—the implementation of the clinical nurse leader (CNL) role. The CNL is a master's-prepared nurse who possesses the competencies necessary to address the lateral integration of care delivery in collaboration with other healthcare disciplines and leads PI initiatives designed to improve patient care outcomes such as HAPU and CAUTI rates at the microsystem (unit) level (American Association of Colleges of Nursing, 2007). A medical–surgical unit was selected as the target site for CNL role introduction, and a new graduate CNL (who had been a staff nurse on the designated unit) was selected. Although no statistically significant improvements were found within the first year of the CNL role implementation, clinical significance during the first year and zero unit HAPU and CAUTI rates were achieved one year after role implementation. Nursing leaders should consider the implementation of the CNL role as a strategy to foster interdisciplinary collaboration and clinical outcome improvements at the microsystem level. As noted previously, a healthcare facility's microsystem improvements may favorably impact macrosystem patient care outcomes and overall improvements to care delivery.

## Reflection Questions

1. Consider a unit/organization and the Institute of Medicine's Triple Aim objectives. What are the priority clinical outcome improvement projects in the area? How and why were they selected?
2. Reflect upon an improvement conducted on a unit/organization. What was the outcome of the improvement project? How would you describe the effectiveness of those leading the project in ensuring collaboration among the key stakeholders? What did the leaders (formal and informal) do well to encourage team member engagement, and which suggestions do you have to improve full team-member participation?
3. Think about a unit or organization. How would the introduction of a different position such as the clinical nurse leader, clinical educator, or clinical nurse specialist role potentially impact team engagement and interprofessional collaboration to achieve project improvement success and positive outcomes? Which strategies would you use to introduce a new nursing role and ensure interprofessional collaboration and engagement?

## References

American Association of Colleges of Nursing. (2007). White paper on the role of the clinical nurse leader. http://www.aacn.nche.edu/PublicationsandResources/WhitePapers/CNL

American Nurses Association. (2009). *Nursing administration scope and standards of practice*. Silver Spring, MD: Nursesbooks.org.

American Organization of Nurse Executives. (2007). AONE guiding principles for the role of the Nurse executive in patient safety. http://www.aone.org/resources/PDFs/AONE_ GP_Role_Nurse_Exec_Patient_Safety.pdf

Bisognano, M., & Kenney, C. (2012). *Pursuing the triple aim.* San Francisco, CA: Jossey-Boss.

Harris, J. L., Roussel, L., Walters, S.E., & Dearman, C. (2011). *Project planning and management: A guide for CNLs, DNPs and nurse executives.* Sudbury, MA: Jones and Bartlett.

Rath, T., (2007). *Strengths finders 2.0.* New York, NY: Gallup Press.

## CHAPTER SIX

# Making the Case for a Project: Needs Assessment

*Carolynn Thomas Jones and Linda Roussel*

## Chapter Objectives

1. Identify the primary components of a clinical needs assessment.
2. List the steps to take when completing a needs assessment.
3. Compare a clinical needs assessment and a community needs assessment.
4. Apply principles for project planning needs assessments.

## Key Terms

Business case
Clinical needs
   assessment
Community needs
   assessment

Institutional review board
   (IRB)
Population
Qualitative
Quantitative

Reliable
Replicable
Stakeholders
Transparent
Validity

## Roles

Project leader

Researcher

## Professional Values

Advocacy

Confidentiality

Quality

## Core Competencies

Advocacy
Assessment
Coordination

Data management
Design
Development

Stewardship
SWOT analysis

# Introduction

The identification of a need is the cornerstone for project planning when an organization is starting a new clinical program or a community is considering enhancing existing services. Unmet need motivates the formation of laws, policies, innovative practices, learning, treatment, and health service funding (Harrison, Young, Butow, & Solomon, 2013). This chapter identifies what a **clinical needs assessment** evaluates, answers the question of why one completes a needs assessment, and outlines steps followed when completing the assessment.

The Institute of Medicine (IOM), in its pivotal report *Crossing the Quality Chasm* (2001), identified six specific aims and observable metrics required for the delivery of quality care (**Figure 6-1**). Each of these six aims can provide direction in developing a needs assessment. A healthcare practitioner could apply several of the primary aims in one over-arching project design, or just focus on a single element.

Consider the use of induced hypothermia (IH) care for patients brought to an emergency department (ED) because they have been resuscitated after sudden cardiac death. For emergency departments that have implemented this protocol, it is important to understand how well this program is managing and operating by measuring several of these outcome factors based on the IOM's six aims:

- *Safe:* What percentage of patients who have experienced sudden cardiac death receive IH? What were the mortality rates or negative morbidity rates of this care?
- *Effective:* Is the protocol being carried out correctly? Are patients maintained in a hypothermic state for the correct amount of time? Are they re-warmed at the correct time and in an appropriate manner?
- *Efficient:* How has the ED budget been impacted by the launch of the IH program? How many staff are trained to deliver this care? How has this program affected staffing levels?
- *Timely:* Is the IH being performed rapidly enough (time from admission to ED to IH)?

Figure 6-1   Six aims and metrics for delivering quality care.

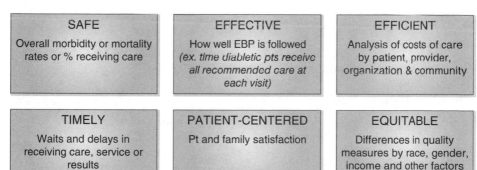

| SAFE | EFFECTIVE | EFFICIENT |
|---|---|---|
| Overall morbidity or mortality rates or % receiving care | How well EBP is followed *(ex. time diabetic pts receive all recommended care at each visit)* | Analysis of costs of care by patient, provider, organization & community |

| TIMELY | PATIENT-CENTERED | EQUITABLE |
|---|---|---|
| Waits and delays in receiving care, service or results | Pt and family satisfaction | Differences in quality measures by race, gender, income and other factors |

*Source:* Data from IOM. (2001). Crossing the quality chasm: A new health system for the 21st century.

- *Patient-centered:* What are the patient and family satisfaction scores, and how do they compare to scores for pre-IH care delivery for sudden cardiac death resuscitation admissions?
- *Equitable:* Are there disparities in how and to whom IH care is being delivered? Are patients with insurance treated differently than those who are uninsured?

These are skeletal examples of how to use the IOM's six aims and metrics for delivering quality care. Applying this rubric to project planning will aid in focusing the development of a robust needs assessment.

For purposes of this chapter, two definitions of a needs assessment are provided. First, the World Health Organization (WHO, 2000) has defined a needs assessment as a tool for project and program planning. Second, a needs assessment may be defined as a systematic review of the way things are and the way they should be (Rouda & Kusy, 1995).

Like any other research methodology, a needs assessment should be **transparent**, **reliable**, and **replicable**. Needs assessments are also dynamic processes. While the assessment may measure "need" or identify "unmet needs" at one point in time to establish a baseline reading, it also provides a means to identify positive or negative shifts, changes, and improvements. Needs assessments can use a combination of **qualitative** and **quantitative** data collection techniques. The steps and considerations for conducting a needs assessment are summarized in **Box 6-1**.

---

**Box 6-1**  Steps to Planning a Needs Assessment

**Step 1: Purpose**
- What is known about the issue?
- What do you want to know?
- What will you do with the information?
- What are your biases?

**Step 2: Population**
- Who is being assessed: A community? A patient population? An institution? A department? A service? A treatment provider?
- What do stakeholders say about this population and approaches to measuring need? (Conduct focus groups or expert panels.)

- Will private health information be collected? How is confidentiality maintained?
- Will an informed consent form be needed?

### Step 3: Method

- Will a survey be used?
- Will it be anonymous?
- Will it be observational?
- Will data collected be quantitative or qualitative?
- Which kind of sampling method will be used?

### Step 4: Instrument

- Are reliable and valid tools being used?
- Will new tools be developed?
- Are questions or queries clearly stated and without bias?
- How will responses be recorded or measured?
- How easy is it to use the instrument?
- Does it include culturally competent language?
- Can results be easily summarized and analyzed?
- Will institutional review board (IRB) review and approval be required? Which type?

### Step 5: Data Collection

- Is there a data management system for collecting and organizing data?
- A data dictionary?
- Key data categories?
- Calculation methods?
- Missing or incomplete data?

### Step 6: Analyses

- What are results?
- What are the assessment's limitations?

### Step 7: Use the results

- Short-term and long-term goals
- Resource allocation

- Summarized findings
- Dissemination plans

DeWitt and Rush (1996) proposed the following four questions to consider when developing the needs assessment:

- Which population has the unmet need, and what proportion of that population will seek services?
- Is there a need for services across several areas?
- What are the types and capacity of services needed to meet the identified needs?
- Can existing services be coordinated to meet needs or improve services?

In 2000, WHO identified three evaluation components that should be considered and/or adopted in the needs assessment process for healthcare services for a given populations:

- Capacity of services in relation to prevalence and incidence of a syndrome or disease in a specific area
- Mix of services required or desired for a syndrome or disease
- Coordination of services in a healthcare delivery system whereby entry, transition, and follow-up occur and are standard practice

## Purpose of Needs Assessment

When assessing needs and capacity within an organization, a SWOT analysis is often used. This assessment identifies the strengths, weaknesses, opportunities and threats impacting an organization at a point in time. SWOT analyses have been used for assessing needs and performing strategic planning in healthcare organizations (van Wijngaarden, Scholten, & van Wijk, 2012). They unpack the dichotomies between external developments (opportunities or threats) and internal capabilities (strengths and weaknesses). A proposed model for SWOT analysis includes a three-pronged approach for its implementation:

- Stakeholder expectations: demands and standards
- Contextual factors: trends and network developments
- Resources: capabilities, people, finance, and means

The goals for a project needs assessment should be clearly identified, and should provide a guide for data collection. The basic components of a needs assessment address the differences between what is known about the idea and what is still unknown. A tenet for all scholarly work, including needs assessment, is "If you do not need to know the answer, then do not ask the question." Therefore, all known and unknown elements and their impact must be assessed to determine their fit with the project. The ultimate goal of any project is to produce usable results that will positively impact functions and deliverables within the organization. If not, then one must ask, "Why did you do it?"

An important element in identification of purpose and need is the identification of biases within the project team, the stakeholders, and the organization as a whole. The needs assessment data can also serve as a guide to project financial impact, justify the allocation of funding by the funding source, and provide support for the **business case**. Business cases are guided by data that validate inefficiencies, the unpredictable nature in organizations, occupational differences, and interdependencies within and across systems.

Another method of assessing quality-associated care and the planning of new projects is to apply the semi-qualitative method developed by Donabedian (1998). This approach is based on three key components: structure, process, and outcomes. Each of these components has direct influence on the others, in a sequential fashion. *Structure* refers to the healthcare setting: personnel (staff expertise), material resources (e.g., electronic health records), and organizational structure (hospital, clinic). *Process* refers to what is done. *Outcomes* refers to health outcomes. Assembling data into these three "buckets" (**Figure 6-2**) can assist in better understanding

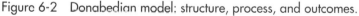

Figure 6-2  Donabedian model: structure, process, and outcomes.

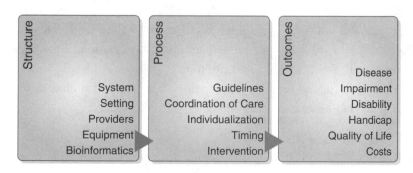

the next steps in identifying key needs and proposed project plans for evolving improvements.

## Population

The population of interest must be described whether the project is focused on an organization, a patient population, or a community. The purpose of the project will guide identification of the population.

Once the population is identified, the project leader and/or team must determine the **stakeholders'** perception of the problem that the project is designed to address. Project team members must collect information from all stakeholders to facilitate an effective problem resolution. For example, identifying similar projects done previously, their outcomes, and any long-term effects will prevent the team from making similar mistakes or duplicating an already effective solution. Stakeholders may include the following groups: (1) patients or those experiencing the need, (2) health and human services providers, (3) government officials, (4) influential people, (5) people whose jobs are impacted by the proposed actions that would result from the assessment, (6) community activists, and (7) affected local businesses.

Population assessment methods can include expert panels, focus groups, surveys, and interviews, among others. The method selected should fit both the population and the project. During this assessment phase, project team members should also determine the level of data that will be collected. For example, if private health information is needed to carry out the project and produce a viable product, then the project team must determine how that information will be collected, stored, and used.

Questions related to maintenance of confidentiality, anonymity and informed consent must be considered. Will data be reported out individually or in aggregate format? How will the research/project team assure security of all information? Inherent in these considerations is "goodness of fit": Do the data fit the purposes of the project and will they yield the desired results? These and other questions provide much context for the project and are also considerations when measuring community needs, as illustrated in **Figure 6-3**.

Reaching informants requires preplanning. It is not uncommon to use more than one method to contact existing and potential stakeholders:

- Social media postings
- Random selection (from telephone directories)

Figure 6-3    Sources and methods for measuring community needs.

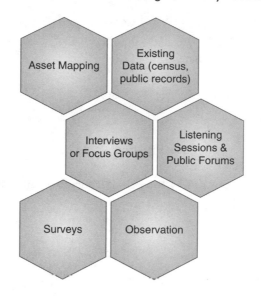

- Mail or email
- Observation of behavior
- Stopping people in public places
- Posters/fliers in public places
- Radio/TV/newspaper advertisement
- Community group outreach
- Personal networking
- Internet surveys (direct to database)

## Methods and Instruments

Project personnel should select the method of data collection and either locate or develop instruments that will best fit the project and the methods. Surveys, for example, are a popular method of gathering information from larger groups. When developing survey questions, it is important to be concise and clear. Questions that fall into categorical (or nominal) level categories should be separated from those that those that fall in ordinal levels.

An example of nominal-level question is

Categorize your highest educational level:
  a. Some high school
  b. High school graduate/GED
  c. Some college
  d. College graduate
  e. Post-baccalaureate

An example of an ordinal-level question would be

Protected learning time (PLT) for ED staff members should be increased to 1 hour per month:
  a. Strongly agree
  b. Agree
  c. Disagree
  d. Strongly disagree

These types of questions can be incorporated into surveys, questionnaires, and interviews.

Other considerations related to methods of data collection include determining whether the data are best captured through a qualitative or quantitative approach. The sampling method to be used is another important component. Samples must be representative of the population and must be sufficient in number to support the findings.

In any project, there is always the possibility of uncovering potential problems in an organization at the micro, meso, or macro level when one is completing a needs assessment. Loo (2003) proposed two methods that organizations may consider using when such problems or issues are identified: an issues analysis chart and an issues impact assessment. An issues analysis chart assists in describing the problem, its impact, and required actions. It complements an issues impact assessment by identifying how the problem(s) may become a barrier to initiating the project and which negative impacts may arise if the problems occur as the project is being completed.

Oliva and Rockart (1997) suggested three other considerations to be taken into account when an organization is conducting a clinical needs assessment: (1) inter-program complementarities, (2) inter-program competition, and (3) interactions among and between programs and services. First, whether or not a project or program was successfully implemented and sustained, organizations must assess how previous projects and programs might have benefited the current endeavor. It is important to determine if tools can be used again or modified for future use. Moreover, if shifts in knowledge, organizational culture, performance, or attitudes occur, those shifts should be measured. Second, organizations should assess the benefits or challenges associated with inter-program competition. Conflicts across programs or competitive programs can become barriers rather than facilitators of the organization's mission, vision, and purpose. Barriers can result in fragmented roles and performance outcomes and ultimately erode employee motivation, resulting in a domino effect of mounting cynicism and deterioration of management's leadership. Finally, organizations must consider the interactions within and between programs and services and examine each program's contributions to the overall success of each unit, the broader organization, and quality of care that will follow.

The IOM (1999) suggests that problems associated with quality of care can be organized into the three categories illustrated in **Figure 6-4**. Underuse, overuse, and misuse may stem from clinical guidelines, policies, equipment, staffing, informatics, authority, funding sources, and many other elements that are at play in structuring and managing a healthcare facility in acute care, long-term care, ambulatory care, or community care.

An example of underuse may occur with electronic medical record data. Nurses and staff who input data into electronic medical records spend a tremendous amount of time on this task. Some of those data are redundant, however; other data are not accessed or used on a routine basis to deliver care. As a consequence, the time spent documenting in the electronic record may not correspond directly to those data's ultimate utility.

Figure 6-4    Three categories for healthcare quality.

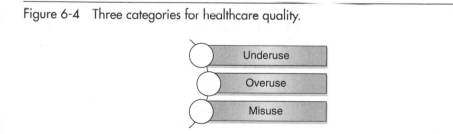

Another example is "work-arounds." Nurses often use "work-arounds" to facilitate the daily activities involved in performing their jobs. For example, some may employ personal mobile devices that aid in getting the job done, but which may be a violation of institutional policy and could jeopardize patient privacy. Such "work-arounds" may represent overuse or misuse issues that impact quality performance and care.

Innovative and creative problem solving can lead to improvements in care delivery; however, it is important to collect data on the utility and risks/benefits of such initiatives. In doing so, it can be useful to consider the underuse, overuse, and misuse issues that are observable and measurable in the organization. Closing gaps in those areas can have a strong positive impact on both quality care and cost savings. The needs assessment is a first step toward planning a project that can address those gaps.

# Human Subject Protections and Institutional Review Board Requirements

The protection of human subjects and adherence to research regulations require an understanding of the subtle differences between quality improvement activities and clinical research. It is especially important to determine if there is a need for informed consent, including the requirement for **institutional review board (IRB)** review and approval. Some may question whether IRB approval is necessary when quality improvement processes and quality assessments are the foci. That argument goes like this: "Since the IRB is predominantly focused on the ethical conduct of research, why should quality improvement projects be reviewed by the IRB? After all, quality improvement is not research."

The response to this argument is that IRB approvals may be necessary for both patient welfare and institutional regulatory adherence. Patients are the focus of quality improvement, process improvement, and research projects, and therefore their rights must be protected (Speers, 2008). Similarly, **community needs assessments** can impact individuals and populations; thus, protection is warranted for communities as well. Moreover, failure to obtain IRB approval can lead to institutional fines and disqualification of the research by federal authorities.

Quality improvement and clinical research share similar aims and are often intermingled. As a consequence, it is sometimes difficult to distinguish between a quality improvement effort and a research effort. Because regulations and bioethical guidelines have evolved, it is important to rely on current requirements when addressing this issue, rather than on comments and opinions of persons who may not currently be knowledgeable about these requirements. In each case (i.e., a quality improvement effort and a research effort), the project leader may formulate a hypothesis (research question or problem statement), determine risks and benefits, and measure outcomes. IRB approval should always be secured prior to any data collection. The type of IRB approval needed will depend on the organization or institutional policies and federal regulations.

Assessments can sometimes cross into the gray zone of "research" based on their level of intensity. For instance, along the continuum between research and direct patient care are various levels of assessment and activity such as quality improvement research, evidence-based practice studies, comparative effectiveness studies, and quality improvement activities. Examples of the various types of healthcare research are illustrated in **Figure 6-5**. This topic is covered in more detail in the chapter *The Institutional Review Board Process.*

Figure 6-5   Types of healthcare "research."

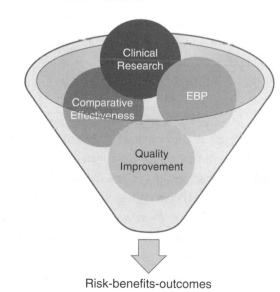

Risk-benefits-outcomes

## Instruments

The **validity** (Does the instrument measure what it is designed to measure?) and reliability (Does the instrument measure the concepts/constructs consistently in different settings, populations, or projects?) of an instrument are integral in determining the usefulness of the project outcomes. If existing tools are available that fit the project, the project team must determine the validity and reliability of those instruments. Traditionally, the validity and reliability of an instrument are described in the original and subsequent research studies that were used to establish them.

If instruments exist but must be altered, the project team must contact the author(s) of the tool and seek permission to use and modify it. Once modified, the instrument must be subjected to procedures to establish the validity and reliability of the modified sections.

If an instrument does not exist that will effectively measure the concepts and constructs of the project, then the researcher or project team may develop a new instrument for use with the project. All researcher- or project team–developed instruments must have their validity and reliability established. Most research texts provide a clear description of the processes and procedures involved in establishing validity and reliability. The reader is encouraged to review such a text for further discussion of this topic.

Instruments must be applicable to the project, expedient, and easy to use. These characteristics are essential not only in collecting data, but also in collating, analyzing, and summarizing the data and disseminating the findings.

## Data Collection

Whether the research or project is large or small, a data management system for collecting and organizing data will be helpful. Data management systems can be quite simple. All that is needed is a mechanism to track the sample involved in the project with regard to where members of the sample are in the process. All team members can use this data management system to determine where each participant is with regard to stage of recruitment, informed consent, data collection, and other stages, and can readily see which data points remain to be collected. The grid shown in **Figure 6-6** is a simple method of managing key data categories.

Figure 6-6   Data collection grid.

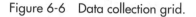

| Participant ID number | Informed Consent | Instrument 1 | Instrument 2 | Data Input Complete |
|---|---|---|---|---|
| | Date Out/Received | Date Out/Received | Date Out/Received | |

A data dictionary or glossary is another useful tool, especially if different members of the team are involved with collecting, categorizing, and entering data. Internal consistency of team usage will facilitate "clean" data collection and entry. Further, consistency in data collection will greatly ease data retrieval and analysis.

The final steps in data collection are determining consistent calculation methods and retrieving missing or incomplete data. Preliminary planning as to how partial and incomplete responses will be incorporated in the findings will assist with these processes.

## Analysis and Use of Findings

Once the data have been collected, they must be analyzed and applied within the organization/system. Any findings must be clearly described and linked back to the original short- and long-term goals and objectives of the project.

Once findings are published, at least internally, resource allocation processes for full implementation can begin. Dissemination of findings to a broader audience will be directly linked to organizational goals and objectives. At this point, the current study and project are considered to have ended, and another problem identification and needs assessment cycle begins.

## Summary

- Needs are the cornerstones for project planning.
- Clinical needs and community assessments provide the rationale and support for the project's business case.
- A series of steps is followed when completing a clinical needs assessment and a community needs assessment.

- A variety of tools can assist the project team when completing a needs assessment.
- Institutional review board approval may be required for projects, especially when the data will be disseminated beyond the organization. Approval is also suggested for internal system data dissemination in support of human subjects' protection.

## Reflection Questions

1. Which elements are part of successful clinical needs assessments and community assessments?
2. What should be considered before beginning the IRB approval process?

## References

DeWitt, D. J., & Rush, B. R. (1996). Evaluation program plan. http://www.springerlink.com/index/UN5V64N5554LO48W8

Donabedian, A. (1988). The quality of care. How can it be assessed? *Journal of the American Medical Association, 269*(12), 1743–1748.

Harrison, J. D., Young, J. M., Butow, P. N., & Solomon, M. J. (2013). Needs in healthcare: What beast is that? *International Journal of Health Services, 43*(3), 567–585.

Institute of Medicine (IOM). (1999). *To err is human.* Washington DC: National Academies Press. http://www.iom.edu/Reports/1999/To-Err-is-Human-Building-A-Safer-Health-System.aspx

Institute of Medicine (IOM). (2001). *Crossing the quality chasm: A new health system for the 21st century.* Washington, DC: National Academies Press. http://www.iom.edu/Reports/2001/Crossing-the-Quality-Chasm-A-New-Health-System-for-the-21st-Century.aspx

Loo, R. (2003). Project management: A core competency for professional nurses and nurse-managers. *Journal of Nurses in Staff Development, 19*(4), 187–193.

Oliva, R., & Rockart, S. (1997). Dynamics of multiple improvement efforts: The program life cycle model. http://www.systemdynamics.org/conferences/1997/paper166.htm

Rouda, R. H., & Kusy, M. E. (1995). Needs assessment: The first step. http://alumnus.caltech.edu/-rouda/T2_NA.html

Speers, M. A. (2008). Editorial: Quality improvement: Research or non-research? AAHRPP perspective. *Association for the Accreditation of Human Research Protection Programs, Advance, 5*(2), 1–2.

Van Wijngaarden, J. D. H., Scholten, G. R. M., & van Wijk, K. P. (2012). Strategic analyses for healthcare organizations: The suitability of the SWOT-analysis. *International Journal of Health Planning and Management, 27*, 34–49.

World Health Organization (WHO). (2000). Needs assessment: Workbook 3. http://whqlibdoc.who.int/hq/2000/WHO_MSD_MSB_00.2d.pdf

# Case Exemplar

## Applications for Project Planning and Management in Antimicrobial Stewardship

Core elements and guidelines for a hospital-based antimicrobial stewardship (AMS) program have been described by the Centers for Disease Control and Prevention (CDC, 2014). The impact of antibiotic resistance continues to rank as one of the rising unmet medical needs. "The CDC estimates that more than two million people are infected with antibiotic resistant organisms in approximately 23,000 deaths annually" (p. 3). Moreover, antibiotic prescribing is inappropriate in 20% to 50% of such prescriptions and is contributing to the rising levels of resistance (**Figure 6-7**).

While the primary goal of AMS programs is to improve patient care and public health, a by-product of implementing and tracking these measures is huge financial savings to institutions and the healthcare enterprise. The aim is to use the correct agent, correct dose, and appropriate duration of dosing for desired outcomes in cure or prevention, minimization of toxicity, and prevention of development of resistant organisms. Institutional costs of implementing an antimicrobial resistance program (whether in an inpatient or ambulatory setting) are minimal compared to the resulting

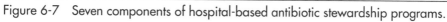

Figure 6-7    Seven components of hospital-based antibiotic stewardship programs.

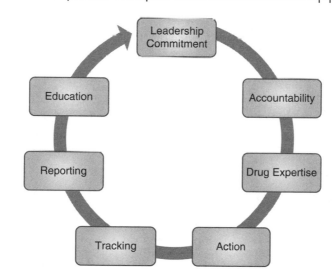

health and financial savings. Building and maintaining sustainability in managing an AMS program is, therefore, an essential challenge for healthcare organizations.

Supporting a business case for ongoing measures requires continuous assessment of need, impact, and resource requirements. Manning (2014) discusses the urgent need for nurse practitioners (NPs) to lead AMS programs in ambulatory care settings and estimates that NPs in those settings write an average 19 prescriptions per day, many of which are for antibiotics. Bedside nurses and infection control nurses have an increasing role in every aspect of AMS.

Project planning and management of a variety of facets of AMS are ripe for advanced practice nurse involvement, whether as a clinician, a nurse executive, or a program manager. After developing a focused approach for problem identification in AMS, the NP should consider how to assess needs from clinical, pharmaceutical, financial, and resource perspectives. A key challenge in such a huge undertaking will be to focus attention on one population, specific organisms, or specific settings, for instance, so as to affect that critical issue positively and bring the project to fruition. Electronic medical record searches based on ICD and CPT coding and use of resources like the Premier Database (www.premierinc.com) are informatics-based approaches that can streamline assessment mechanisms to build a case for project planning and management and offer methods of tracking outcomes.

# ■ CASE STUDY 1

## Project Planning Opportunities Using Case Findings

A 58-year-old woman was driven to a community hospital ED at 0230 by her 84-year-old mother, with complaints of severe epigastric abdominal pain that is reported to be a "15" on a 10-point pain scale. The pain is "constant, but comes in intense waves." The patient, who is a nurse, states, "This is not a typical stomach issue like virus or flu. Something is wrong. I am worried I have some sort of an acute abdomen. Something is not right."

On assessment, the patient has low-grade fever, a heart rate of 110, and a normal blood pressure (110/60 mm Hg); she appears to be in distress. Beyond vital signs, no other physical assessment is performed. The patient denies vomiting and diarrhea. Medical history reveals current medications: Prilosec (for chronic heartburn secondary to hiatal hernia), Zocor, and ramipril (for mild hypertension).

Four weeks prior, the patient had begun treatment with azithromycin for culture-proven *Mycoplasma* pneumonia at a local free-standing acute care facility. Because her symptoms persisted after 10 days, she was prescribed a course of levofloxacin; however, no second culture was obtained. She was sent for an abdominal computed tomography (CT) scan with contrast within 3 hours of arrival and afterward began vomiting. The CT scan was negative. The patient was sent home with a probable diagnosis of "stomach bug" and was given a prescription for ondansetron and pain medication. Once home, the patient began to have diarrhea and continued to vomit. Her stomach pain remained extreme, and she was unable to sleep, maintaining a stressed guarded position. She called a neighbor who was a gastroenterologist, who suggested she go to a different ED immediately.

After presentation to the ED, the patient was admitted to a triage room. Because of her weakened state, extreme pain, and light-headedness, an EKG was performed, which was negative for signs of cardiac ischemia. An abdominal ultrasound was performed and was negative. She was again sent home with a tentative diagnosis of "stomach flu." Her nausea and vomiting persisted, however, and she reported having diarrhea.

On day 4, she pulled some strings and obtained an infectious disease consultation at a local academic medical center outpatient clinic, bringing a stool sample. Because she was taking a proton-pump inhibitor (Prilosec) and had prior antibiotic exposure, the patient was concerned that her continued stomach pain and issues were related to *Clostridium difficile* infection, a condition in which bacteria overgrowth releases toxins that attack the lining of the intestines; it can lead to peritonitis and death after structural ruptures. The infectious disease physician thought the diagnosis was possible, but not probable, given the patient's age and lack of apparent autoimmune disorder. He prescribed metronidazole to be taken for 2 weeks but told her to hold off filling the prescription until stool culture results were confirmatory.

After 3 days, the patient was called and told to begin taking Flagyl—her stool cultures were positive for *C. difficile*. If her symptoms resolved, the patient was to commence high-dose probiotic therapy. If her symptoms did not resolve, she was eligible to consider enrollment in a study protocol using fecal microbiota transplant (FMT). Ultimately, her symptoms subsided with the single 14-day course of metronidazole.

## Nursing Implications

*C. difficile* infections affects 500,000 Americans each year, mostly in hospitals and long-term facilities; however, as many as 36% of those cases are community acquired. Risk factors in community-acquired cases include antibiotic use, use proton-pump inhibitors, and lung infections.

## Case Study Issues

Consider opportunities for project planning and management for community-acquired *C. difficile* infections based on this case study.

- The patient's medical history revealed risk factors for *C. difficile* infection.
- The second round of antibiotics for mycoplasma pneumonia may have been unnecessary.
- Medical staff at two local hospital EDs demonstrated lack of knowledge about *C. difficile*.
- Stool cultures were not obtained at either ED visit.
- The patient's persistence in seeking care, intuition about her condition, and use of influence to obtain an infectious disease consultation resulted in correct assessment and diagnosis; most patients lack this knowledge

and self-advocacy and require advocacy on their behalf by healthcare practitioners.

- The infectious disease physician followed an AMS program by awaiting culture results before commencing Flagyl therapy.
- Probiotic therapy is essential for restructuring normal bacterial flora in the gut.
- The highly contagious *C. difficile* infection requires home-based measures to reduce reinfection or spread of infection to elderly or otherwise compromised persons. All underwear and towels must be washed in hot water with bleach. All surfaces must be washed down frequently with bleach. Avoid sharing bathrooms, if possible. Strict hand washing should be observed.

# ■ CASE STUDY 2

## Using Tools to Meet Patient Needs

Intensive care nursing is fraught with daily challenges in addressing the clinical needs of patients with high acuity and managing diagnostic and pharmaceutical and technological elements of care. Often lacking is attention to basic oral care needs of patients. Consider the impact of poor oral hygiene in critically ill populations and preventable morbidity outcomes. Translate those outcomes into the financial burden imposed on insured persons, insurers, and the healthcare system.

## Case Study Issues

Review a study published by Yildiz, Durna, and Akin (2013) that assessed the unmet medical needs (oral mucous membranes of intensive care unit patients) and the personal and treatment-related variables that impacted the delivery of oral care.

- Discover the tools used to measure needs and outcomes. How were those data analyzed and presented?
- What might be the next steps in project planning and management based on these findings?
- Which other studies in oral care contribute to these findings?
- Which treatment guidelines exist to support program planning?

## References

Centers for Disease Control and Prevention (CDC). (2014). *Core elements of hospital antibiotic stewardship programs.* Atlanta, GA: U.S. Department of Health and Human Services, CDC; 2014. http://www.cdc.gov/getsmart/healthcare/implementation/core-elements.html

Manning, M. L. (2014). The urgent need for nurse practitioners to lead antimicrobial stewardship in ambulatory health care [Editorial]. *Journal of the American Association of Nurse Practitioners, 26*, 411–413.

Yildiz, M., Durna, Z., & Akin, S. (2013). Assessment of oral care needs of patients treated at the intensive care unit. *Journal of Clinical Nursing, 22*, 2734–2747.

## CHAPTER SEVEN

# Using Findings from the Clinical Needs Assessment to Develop, Implement, and Manage Sustainable Projects

*Linda Roussel, Shea Polancich, and Murielle S. Beene*

## *Chapter Objectives*

1. Describe the steps in using a clinical needs assessment for building the case for value-based projects and their management.
2. Describe the life cycle of a project plan.
3. Identify the anticipated project risks and methods for addressing these risks.
4. Analyze the value and pitfalls of various tools, surveys, methods, measures, and strategies used in developing sustainable projects and within clinical microsystems, mesosystems, and macrosystems.
5. Identify leverage and capacity, and explain their relationship in maintaining project and program efficacy.
6. Describe the stakeholders' role in clinical projects and strategies for their engagement throughout the project life cycle.

## *Key Terms*

| | | |
|---|---|---|
| Agility | Evidence | Metrics |

## *Roles*

| | | |
|---|---|---|
| Decision maker | Leader | Risk anticipator |
| Implementation project manager | | |

## *Professional Values*

| | | |
|---|---|---|
| Accountability | Commitment | Evidence-based |

## *Core Competencies*

| | | |
|---|---|---|
| Assessment | Leadership | Management |

# Introduction

Developing, implementing, and managing a project can be a challenging experience, from moving the original idea to planning, carrying out the project, studying the results, and acting on outcomes. Put simply, these steps put the planned work into an actionable framework. Only an estimated 37% of projects are successful—a low rate (Krigsman, 2015) attributed to the often limited time and resources spent to determine the project's overall value to the system. Understanding how to use a value equation and value proposition statement is essential to any possible success. Without a deep dive into understanding the organization's overall mission and goal, a project may squander resources, deliver poor financial returns, create substandard operating processes, compromise products and services to patients, and reduce stakeholders' returns. Despite improved project management methodologies, software development methodologies, and training in those methodologies, there has not been an appreciable increase in the success rate for project implementation over the past 20 years (Phelan & Stockwell, 2014).

The importance of using findings from a needs assessment to inform the developing, planning, and implementing phases of a project cannot be understated. The role of the implementation project manager is essential to this accomplishment, particularly from an interprofessional, collaborative perspective. When managing projects, it is important to have a leader who possesses strong communication skills, is results oriented, understands organizational dynamics, and is committed to corporate values. A close and mutually reinforcing (supportive) relationship exists between developing, planning, implementing, and monitoring. This chapter discusses the value of collaboration in a project's life cycle and the role of the implementation project manager. A description of a systems change model is provided as an example that can assist readers in answering key questions that support project implementation and sustainability in practice settings.

# Project Life Cycle: Role of the Clinical Needs Assessment

The project life cycle consists of four phases: initiation, planning, execution, and evaluation (Gido & Clements, 2015).

In the *initiation* phase of the project life cycle, the scope, purpose, objectives, resources, deliverables, time scales, and structure of the project are defined. These definitions are guided by the results of a clinical needs assessment. A clinical needs assessment considers information (data) from a variety of sources. These data are quantified—for example, length of stay, cost of a day in the intensive care unit, and infection rates. Qualitative data obtained through interviews, focus groups, and observations can add further depth to the needs assessment. A microsystem analysis using the five P's (purpose, population, processes, patterns, and providers) is a helpful assessment tool for obtaining internal data related to the organization and the larger system. With a thorough microsystem analysis, gaps can be identified—for example, between benchmarks and actual infection and falls rates—and further drilled down through a root cause analysis (RCA) and a failure mode effects analysis (FMEA):

- RCA gets at the core of a complication or problem, and considers all aspects of why a particular work process or patient care intervention has not worked as intended, perhaps leading to a fatal event. This type of analysis is generally done after the adverse advent.
- FMEA is a proactive risk mitigation tool that identifies areas of potential failure and considers the severity and probability that a failure will occur. Hazard scores are then assigned based on the severity and frequency of the misstep (failed action) in the process.

RCA and FMEA are tools and processes that give the project team direction when considering the level of information needed to improve the overall process. Their results, which are considered internal data, are essential in determining the need to move forward to improve quality of work and care delivery. Internal data provide the necessary **evidence** and often baseline information for developing a business case, which often includes solutions and a cost/benefit analysis for each possible action for improvement. The feasibility of any one intervention (or a bundle of actions) should be thoroughly considered to ensure that the solution is realistic and has an acceptable level of risk. A project team is chartered to assure that all aspects of the initial plan (the business case) have been thoughtfully considered, and to collectively step through the process to assure consensus and investment in the project plan's success (Gido & Clements, 2015).

In the *planning* phase, a detailed project plan is created, which will be monitored by the project manager and referred to throughout the life of the project. Such monitoring examines results such as cost and quality of expected outcomes. Particular aspects of the project plan include specific information on resources (staffing, equipment, supplies), finances (cost/benefit analysis, return on investment), quality (benchmarks, dashboard, key indicators for effective outcomes), risks (what could go wrong, and how to mitigate or minimize such events), and deliverables (executive summary, manuscript, presentations). It is important to know what you expect to deliver before the team goes too far into implementing the plan (taking action). Accountability for particular deliverables must be established early on in the planning phase to assure that dissemination of results and sustainability are as important as implementing and evaluating the overall results (Gido & Clements, 2015).

*Execution* involves staying on task when implementing the action plan. The project manager and the team consider monitoring of time (tracking and recording time spent on the various aspects of the plan), cost (under/over budget), quality (indicators, outcomes), change (was there enough preparation in readying the environment for the change?), risks (were strategies taken to minimize risk and eliminate barriers?), buy-in (is there acceptance of the intervention strategies taken?), and communication (does information flow freely, is there transparency in how the project is going?). A communication plan is important to assuring that all stakeholders are kept apprised of the actions taken, any complications or risks mitigated, and success (or failure) in realizing the expected outcomes. Sharing this information is essential to the success of the project and to future dissemination of its learnings, extension of its scope, and sustainability (Gido & Clements, 2015).

*Evaluation* involves reviewing overall project outcomes, performance of the project team, and stakeholder involvement. Did the project deliver the benefits, meet the objectives, produce the deliverables on time and within budget, and use resources wisely? Did the action plan follow the expected pathway (management processes)? Was the project team able to determine key project achievements, failures, and lessons learned to inform future direction? Referring back to the initiation and planning phases, the project team considers how the project performed relative to the description in the business case, objectives (outcomes), quality targets, timelines, budget, and resources. Did the internal and external (research) evidence used to support the interventions (action) work as anticipated? How does this contribute to the larger system? What are the implications for spread and dissemination? Within the overall summary (executive summary), key elements to include are the major achievements (positive effects/ benefits), failures (what did not go as planned), and lessons learned and recommendations (next steps). A successful project management plan and model can inform future projects, serving as a guide (template) for ongoing deliberate work of the project team (Gido & Clements, 2015).

## Planning for Implementation

A successful implementation begins with the creation of an executable work plan. The implementation project manager is responsible for crafting the details of this plan—an activity that includes defining goals, objectives, and strategies; developing a timeline; establishing project milestones; and matching project tasks with resources. During the planning process, it is also important to consider overall aims, goals, outcomes, costs, and budgets simultaneously.

## Developing a Project Charter

Developing a written charter is one method of providing clarity regarding the goals, objectives, and timelines for a project plan. In addition, a charter is a key aspect of improvement in that it establishes the written plan for an improvement intervention and defines the small test-of-change methods that will be used. In health care and specific to improvement teams, the elements of the charter provide the framework or scaffold for the project plan and the improvement team who will be responsible for initiating the plan (Richter & Scudder, 2014).

To create a functional written charter, the first step is to form an interprofessional team whose members will work together cohesively to meet the improvement plan or project goals. A team is formed based on the needs of the project to be completed. The skills of the members selected are those necessary to provide insight into the most efficient and effective methods to meet the project goals.

The team's initial composition may be expanded over time as the project goals and objectives are fleshed out and if additional representation is deemed necessary. However, it is essential that those persons involved in the work be the individuals most directly affected by the work to be accomplished as well as those who have the authority and responsibility to effect change.

Once a team is formed, the members of the group operationally define all aspects of the project plan and establish the written charter. A written charter may be developed using an established template that provides a "checklist" of all essential elements for developing, implementing, and evaluating an intervention or improvement project (Richter & Scudder, 2014). Key elements of a written charter may include items such as a project title that clearly articulates the context of the project, dates of project initiation and completion, a listing of team members who will participate in the project, and executive sponsors and team leaders to address the "demographics" of the project. Other sections of the charter may include, but are not limited to, a methodological framework for completing the project; a section providing data and operational definitions for **metrics** used; a section on literature appraisal and synthesis for concepts relevant to the topic and the interventions envisioned; a section for process mapping and any other analyses performed to provide context or direction for the project (e.g., analyses such as policy assessments and strengths/weaknesses/opportunities/threats [SWOT] assessments); and a defined project plan with numbered "steps," resources needed, timelines (for initiation and completion of steps), assigned accountabilities, interventions, and evaluations for the steps and the overall plan. Additional items that are relevant to the charter may include items such an evaluation and recommendations section as well as a plan for dissemination and sustainability of improvements or interventions.

In summary, the charter should clearly articulate the goals and objectives of the defined improvement effort or project. With a written, clear, well-defined charter, there is less room for ambiguity of goals and interpretation errors of the project plan. Moreover, a clearly defined charter assists in decreasing project scope creep. Therefore, it is recommended that a written charter be clearly defined using some degree of standardization and consistency of elements (Richter & Scudder, 2014).

## Model for Improvement

One methodological framework that may be used in project planning and as the underpinnings of the written charter is the Model for Improvement (MFI; Langley, Moen, Nolan, Nolan, Norman, & Provost, 2009). The MFI provides a strong foundation and plan for any improvement effort or intervention. Using the three guiding questions of the MFI may assist the project team in clearly articulating the goals, aims, and/or objectives of the project:

1. What am I trying to accomplish?
2. How will I know a change is an improvement?
3. Which changes can I implement that will result in an improvement?

These three questions provide clarity of purpose and form the central components for a project plan (Langley et al., 2009).

The initial guiding question is central to providing the goal of the project. What is the overall goal or objective that the group should work toward? Sometimes answering this question is more difficult than one would imagine. Indeed, projects that are broad in scope may have many smaller subprojects that need to be completed before a goal representing a broader perspective may be accomplished. The reverse may also occur. A smaller project may mushroom into one with a broader, more global view of or perspective on a process. For example, a team may form to understand the transfer of a patient through a hospital with a pain pump, but upon better understanding of the elements of the project, the goal may change to become standardizing "pain management processes" throughout a facility. Clearly defining the ultimate goal is central to developing a project plan that will meet that goal.

The second question of the MFI provides the evaluation criteria for the improvement efforts or intervention that is being implemented and tested. It is necessary to provide an analytical assessment of an improvement effort to demonstrate measurable results. Defined measurable criteria are articulated by operationally defining the metrics that will be used to achieve baseline measurements and post-intervention or post-implementation measurements. Operational definitions are necessary to clearly define a numerical measure, as well as the tools or methods used to perform that measurement. For example, when defining a rate for "patient falls," it is necessary to define the term "fall" as well as the means by which the rate will be measured. What are the numerator and the denominator for the rate, and are there specific inclusion and exclusion criteria that should be used? Evaluation of an improvement will guide the process of either disseminating the intervention established or changing the plan and revising the implementation if the goals and objectives set for the improvement are not met (Langley et al., 2009).

The final question in the MFI seeks to define the intervention that will be used to improve the process being evaluated. In this step, the team envisions a change that will lead to an improvement in the outcome defined by the measure or evaluation in the second guiding question. For example, if the team intended to improve the patient fall rate, then an intervention specific to falls would be developed. This may include processes such as developing and implementing a more accurate, evidence-based "falls risk assessment" tool on a nursing unit. The intervention is first defined and operationalized and then implemented and evaluated (Langley et al., 2009).

The three guiding questions of the MFI "set the stage" or provide the foundation for "testing" change that may lead to improving a process. Small tests of change are often accomplished through the use of a plan–do–study–act (PDSA) cycle. The PDSA cycle is the engine for change that one would use to *plan* an improvement effort, *do* or implement the plan, *study* the results of the implemented plan, and *act* upon the results by either disseminating the project or changing the plan and repeating in an iterative fashion. Small test-of-change, PDSA cycles are a method for testing improvement interventions in a systematic and focused manner.

Use of the MFI and PDSA approach may provide standardization of improvement efforts within a project plan, and should be included in the written charter. The articulation and definition of these elements provide clarity for project efforts and may assist in focusing a project or improvement team on the project goals and objectives (Langley et al., 2009).

The project manager leads the team in conducting a SWOT analysis, in which team identifies strengths and weaknesses (internal forces) as well as opportunities and threats (external forces). The strengths and opportunities are positive forces that can be exploited to efficiently implement a project. Weaknesses and threats may hamper project implementation, if they are not considered in light of the overall aims and context of the project. Many organizations simultaneously conduct a needs assessment and a SWOT analysis and then compare findings. The needs assessment focuses on a summary of the following areas:

- Descriptions of the qualitative and quantitative data that support the need for the project
- The costs, resources, stakeholder buy-in, and work requirements necessary for a successful and meaningful project outcome prior to implementation
- Determination of whether needs are strategically aligned with the organization's mission and overall goals

The information gleaned from the needs assessment is pivotal and requires comprehensive consideration prior to planning and implementing a project. In this step, the role of the implementation project manager transitions into that of risk anticipator, assisting project stakeholders in devising a strategy means of overcoming potential barriers. It is best to begin with the end in mind. That is, what is the expectation for quality outcomes when undertaking a project initiative? Lighter (2011), for example, identified the need for stakeholders to consider the value proposition when implementing a project. More specifically, he proposed the following formula to calculate value:

Value = quality/cost

According to Skor (2013), establishing a substantive value proposition is critical to successful companies and projects undertaken to meet operational goals. This step starts the journey from the inception of an idea to completion of the project. Skor defines a value proposition as a positioning statement that outlines the benefits provided for the agent or company and explains how those benefits uniquely address the need. The target market, the problem to be solved, and why this solution is better than the alternatives are other information included in a well-stated value proposition. The creation of a compelling value proposition includes four steps: (1) defining, (2) evaluating, (3) measuring, and (4) building.

In the *defining* step, the team provides the information that determines if the problem is worth solving. Skor (2013) describes the four U's as being significant to defining the value proposition. If the answers are "yes" to the majority of these questions, it is likely that the project planners are moving in the right direction toward a compelling value proposition:

1. *Is the concern Unworkable?* If there were inaction in regard to a real problem, perhaps someone gets fired without addressing the issue, or you lose a major customer, this would likely direct the need to finding a solution. For example, the person who may be fired would likely be an excellent internal champion of the project.

2. *Is fixing the problem Unavoidable?* If regulatory or accreditation issues are on the table, that factor drives fundamental requirements for compliance and accountability issues. Answering "yes" to this question would likely identify the group that should serve as a champion for the project.

3. *Is the concern Urgent?* Is this concern a top priority to the system? Without attention to the issue, would you likely lose market share or other major resources? If the answer is "yes," the corporate suite's attention will likely be drawn to the concern.

4. *Is the problem Underserved?* If there appears to be no (or limited) solution to the problem you want to address, you may be identifying a segment of the market (or white space) that would increase your organization's value. If you answer "yes" to this question, then your company may be primed to increase its market share.

Another tool that Skor (2013) recommends is qualifying the problem as "BLAC and White." BLAC is an acronym standing for Blatant, Latent, Aspirational, and Critical; White refers to the "white space" that the projects capitalize on as an opportunity for growth. Skor notes that concerns or problems that are blatant and critical are more likely to attract attention because they tend to stand in the way of doing business and are more acute than latent or aspirational problems. When a problem is latent, it is generally unacknowledged; aspirational problems are considered optional, and are often the most difficult to consider in a fast-based frenetic market.

The second step, *evaluating,* seeks to determine whether the solution is unique or compelling enough to continue the effort in the planning. Once the problem is defined as critical for pursuing, the team must identify what is unique and compelling about a solution to this problem. Skor (2013) offers a useful approach in the context of the three D's. The three D's provide a thoughtful approach to considering the unique combination of *D*iscontinuous innovation, *D*efensible technology, and a *D*isruptive business model that makes a solution compelling to the team and its target—a possibly skeptical market. A *discontinuous* innovation provides transformative benefits over the status quo by viewing the problem through different lenses. *Defensible* technology encompasses intellectual property that can be protected to develop a barrier to entry and an unfair competitive advantage. *Disruptive* business models can catalyze the growth of the venture by enabling its employees to understand the value and cost rewards. While "faster, cheaper, and better" may also be a useful metric, evaluating the three D's can expand thinking about a potential breakthrough.

Skor's (2013) third step, *measure,* considers the gain/pain ratio of potential adoption of a solution to a problem. This ratio compares the gain that solution will deliver to the target market versus the pain and cost required for the solution's adoption. Skor reports that he looks for nondisruptive innovations—that is, those technologies that offer game-changing benefits yet require only minimal modifications to current processes and systems. Nondisruptive introduction is essential to new projects, because the gains they deliver will be discounted by the risks associated with altering the current system. A successful venture delivers an order of magnitude improvement over the status quo. According to Skor, if you are not able to deliver a 10-fold gain/pain promise, stakeholders and the target market will typically default to "do nothing" rather than bearing the risk of working with you. To overcome this reluctance to change, you will need to assure that your innovation is measurable to a degree that change is notable.

Skor's (2013) final step, *build,* involves moving from defining, evaluating, and measuring to actually creating the value proposition. Skor recommends the following framework for the *building* step:

1. Who are your stakeholders? Your target customers?
2. Who and what are dissatisfied with your current performance?
3. What will this new strategy (product) be?
4. What will be provided? What provides key problem-solving capability?
5. What is unlike your product? What is the product (intervention) alternative?

According to Skor (2013), that the most important consideration is the individual (*you*) that creates the value proposition and carries out the strategies. You, the project planner, are core to *your* value proposition. How do *you* understand and deliver uniquely? Which kind of disruptive business model can *you* bring? Skor describes being true to *yourself* as a thought leader as a means to ensure that *you* will go far.

Inherent in the planning process is the development of an implementation strategy. The implementation strategy is meant to focus on the process from a stakeholder perspective and should be approved prior to execution. The most common implementation strategy is the phased approach for a project (Glaser, 2009). This approach is relatively safe for the organization because it allows the project team members to reassess their progress after each project phase is operationalized. For example, in a project to reduce catheter-acquired urinary tract infections (CAUTIs), phases may include determination of the extent of the problem, use of data to drive urgency to act (magnitude of problem), outcomes to be measured, implementation strategies, and evaluation protocols.

A key document in the implementation phase is the project charter. The project charter is an agreement between the organization providing the service and the stakeholder requesting the service and receiving the deliverables (Lewis, 2005). It includes a comprehensive description of the project, a list of anticipated project team members, and those members' specific roles and responsibilities in the project. Also included in the charter is the level of authority for the project manager and the project outcomes. The project charter outlines the scope and measures of success, and includes formal signatures for project authorization and approval. This process is critical to building consensus on project goals and documents communication between project stakeholders.

For example, a project aimed at reducing CAUTIs on an acute surgical unit might involve the clinical nurse leader (CNL), the infection control nurse, a patient representative, and staff nurses. The CNL may take the lead as project manager, outlining particular roles of each member (e.g., observing how patients' urinary catheters are handled during transport, monitoring the number of catheters inserted and discontinued). Tasks related to setting up communication channels, meeting times, and review tools may also be established and delegated by the CNL. While other team members are intimately involved in the implementation of the project and have an active voice in all project-related measures, the CNL is the project manager, but he or she cannot and should not be expected to produce the project outcomes alone.

Another phase of the project implementation may revolve around the action plan (based on the best available evidence) that delineates particular strategies. The action plan includes the following elements:

- How evidence-based interventions will be used to improve the system (system change) and practice
- The *how* to accomplish the stated purpose
- The collaboration and teamwork required to implement the project, its sustainability, and its relevance to an existing program or mission
- Information flow processes (informatics and technology)
- Interventions that will focus on educating others about the project and means by which the information provided will guide stakeholders throughout the implementation phase and result in the stated project goal/aim
- Descriptions of the theoretical or conceptual underpinnings and their relevance to the overall project and program mission
- How organizational and cultural dynamics will be addressed
- Anticipated impacts that the project will have and explanation of how findings will close gaps identified by the SWOT analysis and needs assessment
- Time-specific milestones

An evaluation phase to measure the success of actions taken is important to determine the efficacy of the plan. An evaluation plan includes the following elements:

- Methods and metrics for evaluating the project
- Timelines and data milestones
- Measurement types that include structure, process, and outcome
- Metrics that gather evidence relevant to stakeholders and the system, are scientifically sound, and are associated with processes that can be modified through reasonable methods and procedures

- Lessons learned, barriers that were overcome during the implementation phase, and strategies used to overcome the barriers that could further inform the project

## Micro, Meso, and Macro Collaboration

Collaboration across organizational stakeholders requires communication, commitment, accountability, and continuity (McElmurry et al., 2009). To ensure that a new initiative is realized to its full potential, stakeholders must see the strategic alignment. Administrative support for a project may enhance successful implementation and sustainability. For example, a project for reducing CAUTIs aimed at reducing patients' discomfort and costs of care serves to advance the mission of the organization. In particular, it addresses the overall mission of quality—that is, safe care. The implementation project manager translates to stakeholders how existing business processes would be improved with project implementation. Project stakeholders (project sponsors, decision makers, and leaders) in a healthcare organization publicly endorsing the project may underscore the importance of the project's purpose.

In terms of the implementation of a project, collaboration with stakeholders is priceless. It is important to involve organizational stakeholders from the beginning, perform intermittent progress checks, be responsive to concerns, and address risks throughout implementation. At the point of implementation, the project manager ensures resource needs are clear and project risks are reviewed and validated. Stakeholder expectations must be managed during implementation through continued focus on the strategic goals of the project (McElmurry et al., 2009). Structure, process, and outcome indicators are continually evaluated to assure that resources are being used efficiently and effectively. Meetings to share progress and lessons learned—for example, actual reductions in CAUTI rates—will further enhance the credibility of the project team's work.

## Communicate, Communicate, and Communicate

In addition to planning and collaboration, the other fundamental element of implementation is communication. The purpose of communications management is to share the right information, at the right time, with the right people, and in the right format. Good communications management requires expending effort on sharing information, which contributes to project success; conversely, lack of information can lead to failure. Most importantly, the project manager must identify the correct target audience for different categories of communications.

Strong communication must be accompanied by mutual trust. Both formal and informal methods can be used to disseminate information. Formal communication methods follow well-defined, systematic procedures, whereas informal communications are casual and more extemporaneous. Weekly status reports containing information about progress and issues are examples of a formal communication tool. Examples of informal communication include voice mail, e-mail, and text messages. An effective and perhaps an efficient method of conveying information within a team is face-to-face conversation.

The implementation plan should be circulated to all stakeholders involved in the project. The implementation project manager must communicate continually to reinforce the messages related to that plan and make sure everyone is ready when implementation begins.

The management of communication is implemented through three essential processes:

- *Identification:* The process of identifying information to be shared, when it should be distributed, who should receive it, and how it should be prepared.
- *Reporting:* The process of collecting and preparing the information.
- *Distribution:* The process of disseminating the information, and for formal communications, storing the information in the project archive.

## Change Management

Change management is possibly the most important factor in the implementation process. For example, when a healthcare organization is adopting a new clinical or financial information system, its business processes will undergo significant changes, so there will be a definite learning curve. The change process must be actively managed. Change management may be led by someone external to the organization, possibly a consultant, and begins at the same time as implementation. The individual or group of individuals charged with handling this task should collaborate with the implementation project manager and project stakeholders to craft a change management blueprint tailored for the organization.

An effective change management technique is for one department to test the new approach before it is rolled out more broadly. In other words, rather than a big-bang start, it is often more productive to begin with one unit or department trying out the project initiative. A staged approach allows the implementation project manager and stakeholders to monitor the initiative at work on a small scale and react to any resulting issues. This steady progression generates confidence and understanding throughout the organization, building buy-in for the project. This gradual process of integration can be replicated with employees as well. They are encouraged to start off slowly and build their knowledge and confidence related to the project initiative.

Faculty members from the University of South Alabama College of Nursing developed a model that visually illustrates the intersecting aspects of a system change project that can assist organizations and students when planning and implementing a project (**Figure 7-1**). Questions are posed for each intersecting aspect that can guide the implementation of the system change project. The intersecting aspects and accompanying questions are presented here:

## Evidence-Based Practice: Incorporates IOM Aims, Models, Levels, Guidelines, and Critical Appraisal

- Is there a model or framework of how evidence is managed?
- Are level(s) identified?
- Is there a critical appraisal mechanism?

## Quality Improvement: Measurable Outcomes and Evaluative Structures

- Is a model/framework plan in place?
- What is the quality improvement process?

Figure 7-1   System change project intersecting aspects.

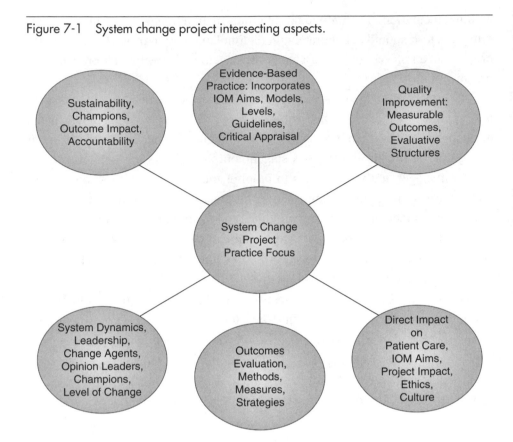

## *Direct Impact on Patient Care, IOM Aims, Project Impact, Ethics, and Culture*

- Are the aims clearly defined?
- What is the direct impact on patient care?

## *Outcomes Evaluation, Methods, Measures, and Strategies*

- Are outcomes defined?
- Are measures to be evaluated identified?
- Are methods to evaluate outcomes defined?

## *System Dynamics, Leadership, Change Agents, Opinion Leaders, Champions, and Level of Change*

- Is there a conceptual/theoretical framework identified?
- Is it integrated into the project plan?
- Which system(s) are to be changed?
- Who are the change agents? Opinion leaders? Change champions?
- Is this an incremental change? Transformational change? How do you know?

## *Sustainability, Champions, Outcome Impact, and Accountability*

- Do long-term plans exist?
- Which plans are in place to maintain sustainability?

## Resistance to Change Is a Reality—Embrace It

Training and education play an important role in overcoming resistance in the adoption of new organizational initiatives. Research has revealed that adult learners have the capability to grasp new information early in the implementation phase of a project (Bond, 2006). The implementation project manager must collaborate with educational resources within the organization to develop training materials in the planning process of this project. Equally important is the support of decision makers and leadership in providing these resources to support project efforts.

## Post-Project Monitoring and Evaluation

Projects should be continuously evaluated for quality and appropriateness. Adjustments can then be made at the time of discovery, instead of waiting until the end of project implementation (Kitzmiller, Hunt, & Sproat, 2006). With such an approach, the project may have more minor, smaller adjustments instead of larger, more costly swings in project scope and direction.

Post-implementation reviews can be conducted to identify value achievement progress and the steps still needed to achieve maximum gain. It is extremely rare for healthcare organizations to revisit their investments to determine whether promised value was actually achieved (Glaser, 2009). Some organizations believe that once the implementation is over and the change settles in, value will automatically be achieved (Glaser, 2009). In reality, it is wise for healthcare organizations to conduct reviews of projects periodically to evaluate progress.

Post-implementation reviews support the achievement of value by signaling leadership interest in ensuring the delivery of results, identifying the steps to ensure value, and reinforcing accountability for results. The reviews also answer questions such as the following:

- Which goals were expected to be met at the time the project was approved?
- How close has the organization come to achieving those project goals?
- How much has the organization invested in the project, and how does it compare with the original budget?
- If the organization had to implement the project again, what would it do differently?

Monitoring is an important component of the implementation phase to ensure that the project is implemented per the schedule. It is a continuous process that should be put in place before project implementation starts. Monitoring activities should be executed by all individuals and institutions that have an interest (stakeholders) in the project. To efficiently implement a project, the people planning and implementing it should plan for all the interrelated stages from the beginning. Metrics are also important to ensure that activities are implemented as planned. They help the implementation project manager measure how well he or she is achieving project milestones and goals. As such, the monitoring activities should appear on the work plan and should involve all stakeholders. If project activities are not going well, arrangements should be made to identify the problems as early as possible so that they can be corrected.

Organizations should benchmark their performance in achieving value against the performance of like organizations (Glaser, 2009). These benchmarks may focus on process performance, using data to inform activities ranging from resource allocation to instructional practice. Stakeholders, especially project sponsors, should understand the accountability they have for the successful completion of the project. There should be an agreed-upon set of metrics that will be used to track value delivery. These metrics should be complement the metrics used to evaluate project implementation.

## Project Implementation Challenges and Risks

Many potential challenges and risks may arise in the development, planning, and implementation of projects. Some of the common ones include funding and the management of stakeholders. If numerous stakeholders will be directly involved in the project, at least some political challenges will undoubtedly be encountered. Another frequent implementation challenge is the lack of communication among stakeholders, leadership, and the implementation project manager. Such miscommunication creates divergence in perceptions of critical initiatives that have great potential to benefit a healthcare organization, which in turn could lead to quality and safety risks.

Some common reasons for project implementation failure are poor communication with leadership and stakeholders, organizational resistance to change, scope creep, lack of project ownership and champion, and shifts in organizational priorities. The recommended approach for achieving implementation success is the incorporation of **agility** into the project process (Kitzmiller, Hunt, & Sproat, 2006). Agility is a concept that encourages flexibility, adaptation, and continuous learning as a part of the implementation process. The agility process accepts the complexity of a problem and addresses it through frequent inspection, responding with a flexible approach of constant adaption (Kitzmiller et al., 2006). Agility considers the complexity of the problems faced in the current healthcare environment and enhances traditional implementation techniques.

## Summary

- Implementation is the final process of moving the solution from development to production status.
- Successful implementation begins with an executable plan.
- SWOT analysis and needs assessment are critical to successful project implementation.

- Project charters identify outcomes that can be tracked.
- Collaboration requires communication among and between all stakeholders.
- A systems change project considers several aspects that impact practice outcomes.

## Reflection Questions

1. What are two aspects of project planning that will assure success? Compare them to situations in daily practice.
2. Which factors should be considered when dealing with external forces and barriers that can impede project implementation?
3. Consider a project that you have implemented. Which strengths, weakness, threats, and opportunities did you identify when implementing the project?

## References

Bond, G. E. (2006). Lessons learned from the implementation of web-based nursing intervention. *Computers in Nursing, 24*(2), 66–74.

Gido, J., & Clements, J. P. (2015). *Successful project management* (6th ed.). Boston, MA: Cengage Learning.

Glaser, J. (2009). A strategy for ensuring a project delivers value. *Healthcare Financial Management, 63*(7), 28–31.

Institute of Medicine (2013). U.S. health in international perspective: Shorter lives, poorer health. https://www.iom.edu/Reports/2013/US-Health-in-International-Perspective-Shorter-Lives-Poorer-Health.aspx

Kitzmiller, R., Hunt, E., & Sproat, S. (2006). Adopting best practices: Agility moves from software development to healthcare project management. *Computers in Nursing, 24*(2), 75–82.

Krigsman, M. (2015). CIO analysis: Why 37 percent of projects fail. http://www.zdnet.com/article/cio-analysis-why-37-percent-of-projects-fail/

Langley, G. J., Moen, R. D., Nolan, K. M., Nolan, T. W., Norman, C. L., & Provost, L. P. (2009). *The improvement guide: A practical approach to enhancing organizational performance.* (2nd ed.). San Francisco, CA: Jossey-Bass.

Lewis, J. (2005). *Project planning, scheduling, and control.* New York, NY: McGraw-Hill.

Lighter, D. E. (2011). *Advanced performance improvement in health care.* Sudbury, MA: Jones and Bartlett.

McElmurry, B. J., McCreary, L. L., Park, C. G., Ramos, L., Martinez, E., Parikh, R., Kozik, K., & Fogelfeld, L. (2009). Implementation, outcomes, and lessons learned from a collaborative primary health care program to improve diabetes care among urban Latino populations. *Health Promotion Practice, 10*(2), 293–302.

Phelan, B., & Stockwell, C. (2014). Are your projects delivering business value? http://www.brighthubpm.com/project-planning/128738-are-your-projects-delivering-business-value/?cid=parsely_rec

Richter, L., & Scudder, R. (2014). What is a project charter? http://www.brighthubpm.com/project-planning/5161-what-is-a-project-charter/

Skor, M. (2013, June 14). Four steps to building a compelling value proposition. *Forbes,* http://www.forbes.com/sites/michaelskok/2013/06/14/4-steps-to-building-a-compelling-value-proposition/

# Case Exemplar

## ■ CASE STUDY 1

### LPN-BSN: An Innovative Articulation Model

*K. Michele Lyons*

## Background

The Patient Protection and Affordable Care Act, aging of the U.S. population, and the nursing faculty shortage will all contribute to the expected nursing shortage in the United States. This shortage, in conjunction with the identified need by the Institute of Medicine (2013) for seamless transfer opportunities to allow nurses to enhance their education, prompted the development of an interagency collaborative project between a community college and a four-year university. This project will provide students with an alternative method to enter the workforce so as to meet the needs of the nursing shortage as well as provide students with opportunities to further their education.

This interagency collaborative project was modeled after an existing partnership between the community college and the university. Students who require remediation or do not meet the university's admission requirements are admitted into the program. The courses are offered through the community college and are held on the university campus. Once the student has met the program's requirements, the student seamlessly transfers to the university to continue his or her education. The results of this program have demonstrated that students are more likely to successfully transfer when the classes are held on the university's campus and a clearly outlined matriculation plan has been developed.

## Objectives

The purpose of this project was to develop and implement an accelerated LPN program to increase the nursing workforce and provide a seamless transition to a bachelor of science in nursing (BSN) program. The program outcomes were intended to increase the nursing workforce by developing graduates from an accelerated program who are as academically successful as their traditional counterparts and have the same professional attributes as their traditional counterparts.

## Methods

The accelerated LPN program began in January 2014 and was expected to produce graduates in December 2014. The students are attending classes on the university campus and being exposed to information about matriculation into BSN opportunities at the university as well as the advantages of gaining a BSN for future career advancement. These students were required to have completed specific general education coursework from a four-year university prior to being admitted.

## Results

Demographic data, including preadmission test scores, are being collected for descriptive purposes. Academic performance will be measured using the following outcomes: National Council Licensure Examination for Practical Nurses (NCLEX-PN) scores, Assessment Technologies Institute Comprehensive Indicator scores, and final grade-point averages. The Nurses Professional Values Scale–Revised (NPVS-R), derived from the American Nurses Association's *Code of Ethics for Nursing,* is being utilized to assess the students' ethical values (American Nurses Association & Fowler, 2008). The expectation is that no difference will be found between the accelerated and traditional LPN students' academic performance and ethical values.

## Conclusions

The success of this program will potentially impact nursing education and build a stronger, more diverse workforce. Nursing students should have access to advanced career opportunities within an academic system that allows seamless transfer opportunities.

## Reflection Questions

1.  How was the need determined to initiate this innovative educational program?
2.  Who were the major stakeholders?
3.  How was the project conceptualized?
4.  How were the program outcomes developed?

## References

Institute of Medicine. (2010). *The future of nursing: Leading change, advancing health.* Retrieved from http://books.nap.edu/openbook.php?record_id=12956&page=R1

American Nurses Association, & Fowler, M. D. M. (2008). *Guide to the code of ethics for nurses: Interpretation and application.* Silver Spring, MD: American Nurses Association.

## CHAPTER EIGHT

# Role of Information Technology in Project Planning and Management

*James L. Harris and Todd Harlan*

## *Chapter Objectives*

1. Describe the importance of information technology as an enabler when assessing needs and planning evidence-based clinical projects in today's healthcare environment.
2. Identify key stakeholders, partnerships, and their respective roles in developing information technology that supports clinical projects, enterprises, and their management.
3. Examine the significance of key information technology core competencies and skill sets for successful project plans and management in a global society.
4. Explain the value of linking projects to information systems for enhanced functionality, data conversion, and data utility.
5. Examine the role of data integrity, security, protection of human subjects, and regulatory agencies within the context of planning projects and their management.

## *Key Terms*

Clinical enterprise
Data integrity
Human subjects'
    protection

Information
    management
Information
    technology

Security
Stakeholder
Privacy
Value

## *Roles*

Educator
Leader

Partner

Team member

## *Professional Values*

Efficiency
Integrity

Performance
Privacy

Quality

## *Core Competencies*

Communication
Design

Information technology
    knowledge

Management

# Introduction

The advent of the Patient Protection and Affordable Care Act, also known more simply as the Affordable Care Act (ACA), represents the largest change to the U.S. healthcare system since the genesis of the Medicare and Medicaid programs in 1965 (Institute of Medicine [IOM], 2001, 2011). The U.S. healthcare system has experienced and will continue to undergo numerous changes as the ACA matures and more Americans seek care. How the healthcare industry responds to the ACA, impending care mandates, reimbursement models, and the information age will be driven by knowledgeable consumers and leaders who are able to make informed decisions. The momentum needed for survival will be shaped by how well and how accurately needs are assessed and evidence-based projects are initiated. Quantum leaps in efficiency and effectiveness will be realized as organizations allow informatics to drive the direction of projects and determine the role that the information specialist will play in the process. However, such projects will be only as effective as the partnership that is built with a transformative clinical project manager.

The clinical project manager must be poised to support the project activities with necessary tools, issue management, and coordination (Gallagher, 2012). Ownership of any clinical project is given to clinical **stakeholders** by reinforcing that it is not an **information technology** or support project, but rather a clinically driven project with interprofessional participation as a cornerstone (Lewis, 2011). Ongoing human activities are needed for data conversion and the spread of knowledge. Otherwise, as projects mature, the identified project aims and outcomes will not be realized. The merits of information technology will also be limited in such unsuccessful projects, and improvements in **value** obtained by consumers, payers, and accreditation agencies will be less than optimal (Lighter, 2011).

# Information Technology as an Enabler for Clinical Project Success

What enables a clinical project's success and its management? While there is no one formula that is guaranteed to ensure the project meets its aims, the use of informatics is a valuable tool in today's evolving technological healthcare environment. Investing in new ways to seize opportunities to mix technology with project ideas is equally important as nurses interact with clinical informatics departments. The potential for all nurses to enhance practice, solve clinical problems, and improve care has paved the way for nursing informatics. The professional nurse of the 21st century will be ineffective without a solid base of informatics, computers, and information technology (Kelly, 2012). Likewise, individuals engaged in clinical projects will experience a similar void if this knowledge base is lacking. Understanding the scope of nursing informatics provides context. It serves as an enabler when identifying needs that structure project aims, guides related processes, and ultimately shapes the outcomes (National Advisory Council on Nurse Education and Practice, 1997). Leveraging the skills of informatics specialists when developing new projects and adopting measurement tools can optimize iterative processes that limit workarounds. Also, the creation of a digital culture for healthcare organizations can be achieved (Morrison, 2011). Informatics and technological advances provide clinical applications that can process transactions with tools for productivity, business strategies, collaboration, and innovations by exploiting unique technological advances (Shane, 1998).

Now we can answer the earlier question: What enables a project's success and its ongoing management? Numerous individuals and organizations have identified multiple enablers that support many projects, programs, and organizational efficacy, and are used daily to improve care (California HealthCare Foundation and First Consulting Group, 2002; DeLaune & Ladner, 2009; Stevens & Staley, 2006):

- Computerized order entry
- Electronic health records
- Mobile communication devices
- Securing messaging and email
- Automated documentation templates and clinical reminders
- Medication administration and management systems

- Evidence-based knowledge and information retrieval systems with remote library and Internet resources
- Quality improvement data collection and data summary systems
- Data mining techniques for sorting large data batches
- Web pages for personalizing information
- Disease surveillance systems
- Computerized data encounter archives

These enablers and their supporting information technology (IT) systems have created multiple opportunities that assist providers daily in responding to patient needs. They serve as milestones whereby IT's ability to facilitate past and future project success and ongoing project management can be measured. Freeing staff from repetitive tasks via IT provides more opportunities for staff to engage with patients and engenders a culture of patient-centeredness.

To maximize each of these enablers and IT systems when planning a project, many considerations must be taken into account and will prove beneficial at steps ranging from the needs assessment phase to completion of the project and dissemination of results. For the purposes of this chapter, two especially important considerations are the organizational mission statement and critical success factors.

As the project is planned, reviewing the organizational mission statement and linking the project focus to the mission can both directly and indirectly prove beneficial in securing buy-in and support. Examples of the benefits from such links may include financial benefits, meeting quality service and patient and/or employee satisfaction objectives, and continuous opportunities for learning and growth.

Critical success factors (CSF) are those elements that must work effectively to ensure high performance within an organization. For example, CSFs are used to prioritize operational initiatives and assist leaders in choosing the most pressing and relevant activities and projects to initiate and support. Again, being cognizant of these factors and linking them to the project and processes will yield positive outcomes.

## Stakeholder and Partner Roles in Information Technology

Identifying and engaging stakeholders continuously during a clinical project is pivotal to that project's success. Similarly, information technology must be an integral part of data retrieval and meaningful use to an organization. As stakeholders participate in a project, whether by engaging in the approval process or by offering encouragement, keeping in mind the need to represent their interests is important to the ongoing phases of any project or **clinical enterprise**. When stakeholders participate, partnerships emerge, ownership is reinforced, and support for the project takes center stage.

An imperative for participation by stakeholders and ongoing partnerships is the commitment and value that information technology development provides and IT's role throughout the project and the organization. The demand for value with any project endeavor will continuously be emphasized, as will the need to invest in value-based IT if gaps in clinical care are to be filled. End users will assist in communicating the value to stakeholders and the utility of supporting all projects, their implementation, and their sustainability in the long term.

As a student or expert project developer considers and plans new projects or redesigns those that may have previously failed, IT investment and partnerships between project managers and IT departments will create a competitive edge for the organization. However, the magnitude of this effect will depend on how well IT systems are designed and their relationships to other business and organizational metrics. As knowledge is generated and spread, and the information generated in terms of local project outcomes is interconnected with national information resources, variability among data will be minimized. Information exchanges will therefore guide clinical and organizational decisions (Sicotte & Paré, 2010). Opportunities for avoiding and managing risk will be created and deleterious errors reduced. The content of information exchanges will be further strengthened as informatics core competencies and skill sets are developed and utilized, and as IT specialists are engaged during all phases of a project.

# Informatics Core Competencies and Skill Sets

In today's global environment and economy, IT has become a thread woven throughout all types of organizations. Whether an individual is directly or indirectly involved in patient care or beginning a clinical project, he or she must be armed with a general knowledge of informatics. The need for organizational and care efficiency, for example, requires healthcare team members to review and mine data so that they can design or redesign care delivery models and productivity. Such activities require competency and skills in informatics, both general and advanced. For those individuals with limited informatics knowledge, knowing where to seek assistance is essential if goals are to be attained. This need resonates with one of the IOM's healthcare professional core competencies (utilize informatics); indeed, its fifth healthcare profession core competency is delineated as the ability to "communicate, manage knowledge, mitigate error, and support decision making using information technology" (IOM, 2003, p. 4). Likewise, the IOM's report *The Future of Nursing* (2011) and the position statement from the Healthcare Information and Management Systems Society (2011) echo the need for nurses to possess informatics competency and skills.

Recognition of the significance of IT core competencies and skills for successful projects and management dates to early work at the University of Maryland that identified three levels of competencies (technical, professional, and advanced) for its multidisciplinary student body (Ball & Douglas, 1989). Grobe's (1988, 1989) seminal work describing informatics competencies for medical students was later modified to create seven levels of informatics competencies for nursing students. **Box 8-1** identifies these seven levels of competencies.

The method used by Grobe made it difficult to confirm that nurses had updated their competencies in this area. Nevertheless, Grobe's work represented a beginning step toward identifying a comprehensive taxonomy of competencies that exist on a continuum ranging from user to modifier to innovator. A further step followed in which a competency grid for each practice domain linked the role functions for each domain (clinical practice, nurse manager, nurse educator, and nurse researcher) with a corresponding range of nursing informatics competencies (technical, professional, and advanced).

| **Box 8-1** | Grobe's Nursing Informatics Competencies for Basic and Graduate Nursing Education |
|---|---|

1. Use basic information-handling tools
2. Independently learn about computers and **information management**
3. Use computer systems and access databases
4. Knowledgeably use systems and specialized databases
5. Perceive new applications
6. Build systems for personal applications
7. Tool building

For decades, healthcare professionals have advanced their care delivery as new competencies have emerged, including those related to informatics. Likewise, multiple vocabularies have been used to classify care. Given that nurses document care on a 24/7 basis, however, there is no single system used in electronic medical records to record nursing care (Cipriano, 2014). Clark and Lang (1992) identified the key shortcoming associated with this practice: "If we cannot name it, we cannot control it, finance it, teach it, research it, or put [it] into public policy" (p. 109). While advancing clinical competencies is necessary to meet care demands, the ongoing development of informatics competencies will be required for successful data management. Educators must provide guided opportunities for students and graduates to develop meaningful projects that are data-driven and evidence-based. This need is clearly apparent when one reviews baccalaureate, master's, and doctor of nursing practice end-of-program competencies (American Association of Colleges of Nursing [AACN], 2006, 2008, 2011).

The challenges of the digital age call for others to perceive roles differently and to express those perspectives in ways that best fit a sociotechnical culture (Porter-O'Grady & Malloch, 2015). This endeavor encourages transformational thinking and action spanning all disciplines and cultures. Meaningful projects that add value and guide quality and the delivery of safe care will be possible with informed users and managers of data as projects are formed, implemented, replicated, and linked to information systems.

## The Value of Linking Projects to Information Systems

From the inception to dissemination of any project, its value must be considered. Value must be attainable and measured to ensure that the resources allotted to a project did, in fact, advance the mission and vision of the organization. Likewise, the value to stakeholders must be measurable and attainable, as they are the end recipients of a clinical project.

Measuring value can be complex and requires use of data from various sources. The data must be informative, relevant, and sensitive to the intent of a project so that a difference is evident in desired outcomes. Meeting this standard requires one to link the project to information systems; otherwise, changing inefficient processes will be more difficult and the value produced may be questionable (Nelson, Batalden, & Godfrey, 2007). Remembering that all healthcare systems are embedded in complex systems, and that all things intersect and are in constant interactions with one another, is important for the success of any project endeavor. Complexity science supports this notion and can inform how value is determined and documented. Linking projects to the correct metrics and information system will aid in measuring the project's value (Porter-O'Grady & Malloch, 2015).

Information systems are the "nervous system" for meaningful projects and can provide the context for how a project benefits practice, education, quality improvement, management, and policy. When planning the project, one must select those metrics that will measure specific outcomes based on the project's aim. Aligning the metrics to the correct information system will isolate the effect of the project based on desired outcomes and allows for greater functionality, conversion, and utility of the data gathered. Conversely, failure to ensure such alignment is a common flaw in the design process. Metrics that effectively measure success extend beyond business and strategic goals and are linked to stakeholders who have a vested interest in the success of any project. Those metrics must be specific and quantifiable (A. Lewis, 2011). To further illustrate this point, consider the example of a clinical success metric identified in **Table 8-1**.

For health informatics projects, Gallagher (2012) identified five phases that provide valuable information for personnel ranging from the novice to the

**Table 8-1**  Clinical Success Metric

| Success Metric | Attainable, Measurable Outcomes from Information System |
|---|---|
| Improved quality, safe, and efficient patient care processes | • Medication order entry errors (pharmacy, medical and nursing services)<br>• Timely signing and verification of emergency verbal orders (medical and nursing services, health information management, pharmacy, and quality improvement) |

expert. First, the *initiation* phase should involve an informaticist when developing project requirements, scope, and vendor contracts and requirements. This can eliminate incongruity between customer expectations and the product. Second, the *planning* phase includes the determination of tasks to ensure design, workflow, and barrier identification. Third, *execution* begins, and the end users of the project are involved as products are tested, adjustments are made, superusers are identified, and education is continuous. The fourth stage involves *monitoring* to ensure all deliverables are met and issues are resolved. Otherwise, the progress of the project can be jeopardized, including the budget. In the final phase, *closing*, all open issues are resolved and any additional modifications completed for a smooth and effective project that will have meaningful use to all involved.

Healthcare-related projects require involvement of a variety of individuals; moreover, to ensure that a project is meaningful, the best available tools must be selected. If quality, safety, efficiency, and continuous improvement are to be achieved with the initiation of any project and its subsequent sustainment, ongoing measurement is pivotal to success. Donabedian (1978) provided an excellent way to characterize medical quality, based on structure, process, and outcome measures. Using Donabedian's model, quality improvement teams consistently use these measures to guide the development of metrics that are linked to data warehouses for easy retrieval.

Lighter (2011) has provided clinically relevant examples using Donabedian's model. Specifically, structure measures describe facilities, staff, and culture of an organization (e.g., number of licensed beds). Process measures relate to the interface between the patient and the provider (e.g., patient satisfaction).

Finally, outcome measures are associated with efficiency and effectiveness of processes, both clinical and business. Accrediting agencies such as The Joint Commission and the Centers for Medicare and Medicaid Services have developed standards and measures using Donabedian's model that demonstrate desirable characteristics such as importance, scientific soundness, and feasibility.

As projects are developed and implemented, keeping the Donabedian model in mind can help team members analyze the value of projects and link it to information systems. Additionally, with the publication of the Meaningful Use Final Rule (*Federal Register*, 2014), projects can be designed to measure the impact of enrolling patients in the clinical patient portal of the electronic medical record. However, ensuring that the integrity of the data is maintained is a mandate that cannot be overlooked.

## Data Integrity, Security, Human Protection, and Use

Health information technology makes it possible for all providers to engage in patient-centered care and to manage care through secure use and sharing of health information. However, maintaining **data integrity**, **security**, and **privacy** is a shared responsibility. It is necessary for all care providers, including students, to receive the necessary education to support safe, secure, and trustworthy practice in the healthcare system. As the care delivery system changes continue to multiply, it is imperative to consider all of the regulatory, technological, and changes that impact practice—including any data that are collected during projects and used to change practice.

Meaningful project planning requires a commitment to both data security and protection of human subjects. This understanding is steered by the sensitivity of the data and the consequences for data compromise. As a quality improvement project or research is executed and data are collected and stored, adhering to the mandates of the Health Insurance Portability and Accountability Act (HIPAA) is essential. This act outlines administrative, physical, and technical safeguards to ensure confidentiality, integrity, and availability of electronic protected health information (Department of Health and Human Services, 2014).

Being mindful of data integrity, security, and **human subjects' protection** must happen in parallel with measures to address ethical, legal, and security issues. While these issues may be primary responsibilities of the organization as outlined in various organizational policies and position descriptions, the shared responsibility of users of that information cannot be dismissed. Numerous safeguards and processes may be established, but individual responsibility in adhering to and respecting them is the key to maintaining the integrity and protection of data and an individual's privacy.

## Summary

- Today's more knowledgeable consumers are demanding accurate and timely data that is easily retrievable and understandable.
- Involving IT specialists in projects can lead to more successful projects.
- Linking projects to organizational mission and critical success factors is beneficial in achieving buy-in, support, and sustainment.
- Interprofessional participation in any project is pivotal to success in today's clinical environment, which is characterized by interconnectivity of activities.
- The professional nurse and other members of the healthcare team of the 21st century will be ineffective without a solid foundation and understanding of information technology and competencies.
- Quality and safety initiatives advance organizational value.
- Information exchanges guide decisions and assist in avoiding information security breaches.
- Information systems are the nervous system of meaningful projects.
- Quality, safety, and continuous improvement will be driven by meaningful use processes and the tools necessary to extract data and spread evidence.
- Data and human protection is essential to avoid ethical, legal, and security issues.

## Reflection Questions

1. What is the role of nurses, project planners, and interprofessional teams in assuring projects align with the ACA?

2. What are three ways a clinical project may engage stakeholders in moving toward meaningful outcomes?

3. How might a project planner outline the steps needed to add value-based project outcomes?

4. Why would interprofessional teams and clinical project developers be concerned with the ethical, legal, and human protection of individuals when considering a clinical project?

# References

American Association of Colleges of Nursing (AACN). (2006). *The essentials of doctor of nursing educator for professional nursing practice.* Washington, DC: Author.

American Association of Colleges of Nursing (AACN). (2008). *The essentials of baccalaureate education for professional nursing practice.* Washington, DC: Author.

American Association of Colleges of Nursing (AACN). (2011). *The essentials of masters education for professional nursing practice.* Washington, DC: Author.

Ball, M. J., & Douglas, J. V. (1989). Informatics in professional education. *Methods of Information in Medicine, 28*(4), 250–254.

California HealthCare Foundation and First Consulting Group. (2002). Report identifies positive impact technology can have on nurse productivity and satisfaction. http://www.chef.org/media/press-releases/2002/report-identifies-positive-impact-technology-can-have-on-nurse-productivity-and-satisfaction

Cipriano, P. F. (2014). What we measure, we can improve. *The American Nurse.* http://www.TheAmericanNurse.org

Clark, J., & Lang, N. (1992). Nursing's next advance: An internal classification for nursing practice. *International Nursing Review, 39*(4), 109 111, 128.

DeLaune, S. C., & Ladner, P. K. (2009). *Fundamentals of nursing standards and practice* (3rd ed.). Clifton Park, New York: Delmar Cengage Learning.

Department of Health and Human Services. (2014). FY 2014 HHS Agency Financial Report. http://www.hhs.gov/afr/

Donabedian, A. (1978). The quality of medical care. *Science, 4344,* 856–864.

*Federal Register.* (2014). 42 CRF Part 495. *Federal Register, 79* (171).

Gallagher, T. (2012). The role of informatics in project management. *HIMSS Clinical Informatics Insights, October,* http://www.himss.org/News/NewsDetail.aspx?ItemNumber=3128

Grobe, S. J. (1988). Nursing informatics competencies for nurse educators and researchers. In H. Peterson & U. Gerdin-Jelger (Eds.), *Preparing nurses for using information systems: Recommended informatics competencies.* 25–40; 117–138 New York, NY: National League for Nursing.

Grobe, S. J. (1989). Nursing informatics competencies. *Methods of Information in Medicine, 28*(4), 267–269.

Healthcare Information and Management Systems Society. (2011, June 17). Position statement on transforming nursing practice through technology and informatics. http://www.himss.org/ASP/index.asp

Institute of Medicine (IOM). (2001). *Crossing the quality chasm: A new health system for the 21st century.* Washington, DC: National Academies Press.

Institute of Medicine (IOM). (2003). *Health professionals education.* Washington, DC: National Academies Press.

Institute of Medicine (IOM). (2011). *The future of nursing: Leading change, advancing health.* Washington, DC: National Academies Press.

Kelly, P. (2012). *Nursing leadership and management* (3rd ed.). Clifton Park, NY: Delmar.

Lewis, A. (2011). Project management. Part II: What works in nursing informatics? http://community.advanceweb.com/blogs/nurses_18/achieve/2011/11/08/project-management-part-ii-what-works-in-nursing-informatics.aspx

Lewis, J. P. (2011). *Project planning, scheduling and control: The ultimate hands-on guide to bridging projects in on time and on budget* (5th ed.). New York, NY: McGraw-Hill.

Lighter, D. M. (2011). *Advanced performance improvement in health care.* Sudbury, MA: Jones and Bartlett.

Morrison, I. (2011). *Leading change in health care.* Chicago, IL: AHA Press Health Forum.

National Advisory Council on Nurse Education and Practice. (1997). *Report to the Secretary of the Department of Health and Human Services: A national informatics agenda for nursing education and practice.* Washington, DC: Health Resources and Services Administration.

Nelson, E. C., Batalden, P. B., & Godfrey, M. M. (2007). *Quality by design: A clinical microsystems approach.* San Francisco, CA: Jossey-Bass.

Porter-O'Grady, T., & Malloch, K. (2015). *Quantum leadership: Building better partnerships for sustainable health.* Burlington, MA: Jones & Bartlett Learning.

Shane, B. (2014). Informatics planning model essential to maximize the effectiveness of IT in supporting program goals. http://www.bpcgallery.com/informatics_planning.htm

Sicotte, C., & Paré, G. (2010). Success in health information exchange: Solving the implementation puzzle. *Social Science & Medicine, 8*(70), 1159–1165.

Stevens, K. R., & Staley, J. M. (2006). The quality chasm reports, evidence-based practice, and nursing response to improve healthcare. *Nursing Outlook, 54*(2), 94–101.

# Case Exemplar

## ■ CASE STUDY 1

### Information Technology: A Valuable Asset for Nursing Informatics Projects

*Todd Harlan*

As technology has evolved, so has nursing informatics. As a leader of an informatics program preparing master's and doctoral nursing students, an overarching theme is coaching students to strengthen their skill sets for success within the industry and organizations. As students matriculate nationally through informatics tracks, project plans and products must be developed that are based on need and evidence to address constantly changing care needs. Outcomes from the developed products will be evaluated both directly and indirectly, as patient care processes are improved and their sustainable value is realized economically.

Students engage in a series of purposeful activities during the process of selecting improvement projects. An informatics needs assessment is central to understanding needs in all organizations, whether at the micro, meso, or macro level. The assessment findings require validation, and teams are often used to perform this task. Of note, more interprofessional team validation of findings has become commonplace with the advent of the electronic medical record (EMR), as it crosses all disciplines. The improvement project plan is then developed based on the assessment findings, industry standards, best available evidence, and stakeholder engagement. Students seek and attain approval prior to progressing with any project, including institutional review board approvals. Throughout the process, venues are abundant for additional student knowledge attainment and synergy of stakeholders as the plan matures and informatics products are created and implemented.

According to McGonigle and Mastrian (2015), the time interval between conduct of research, project outcome dissemination, and clinical translation can be significant. Both patient and system outcomes may be affected adversely by such delays. The issue within many organizations is translating the data that is embedded within the EMR and trying to extrapolate that information for improved patient outcomes.

During their tenure as informatics program leaders, several students have collaboratively developed systems that support an infrastructure aimed at ensuring quality and safety. One example of a value-based collaborative project was a computerized provider order entry (CPOE) system. Such systems allow physicians to capture order information and access other materials that can improve the overall delivery of care and improve patient outcomes. The Healthcare Information Technology for Economic and Clinical Health (HITECH) provision of the American Recovery and Reinvestment Act provided the supporting rationale for the project. This act provides funding to assist with development of a health information technology infrastructure that subsequently improves quality and health care safety (Radley, Wasserman, Olsho, Shoemaker, Spranca, & Bradshaw, 2012). Among the provisions noted were incentive payments to physicians and healthcare facilities to support health IT, including CPOE implementation.

While the CPOE example was specific to one discipline's actions, other projects have focused on issues that directly affect patient care and outcomes. Regardless of the IT project, students tend to identify that the task can be daunting and in some cases very difficult to implement. The constantly changing healthcare landscape, reimbursement issues, and accreditation mandates will require easily extractable data for project success. All student projects are vital to the overall knowledge gained within the theory portions of the informatics track. For the primary instructor, ensuring that students are attaining the stated learning objectives and are assigned to knowledgeable preceptors is essential for success.

Nursing informatics will continue to emerge as a dynamic and value-added asset as care delivery shifts to community settings. The development of integrated IT systems will only expand in the coordination of healthcare delivery. Nurses are in pivotal positions to address this call to action.

# Reflection Questions

1. When assessing the process of an improvement project, what is a central requirement that is crucial to the success of the project? Describe this process, and discuss the advantages and disadvantages if it is not followed.
2. Discuss the premise of data research and dissemination, and explain how the time between these two phases can affect desired outcomes.
3. As discussed in the case study, computerized provider order entry offers many advantages to physicians and other healthcare providers. Expand on these advantages; also discuss any disadvantages that may exist and be constraints to progress.

# References

McGonigle, D., & Mastrian, K. (2015). *Nursing informatics and the foundation of knowledge* (3rd ed.). Burlington, MA: Jones & Bartlett Learning.

Radley, D., Wasserman, M., Olsho, L., Shoemaker, S., Spranca, M., & Bradshaw, B. (2012). Reduction in medication errors in hospitals due to adoption of computerized provider order entry systems. *Journal of the Medical Informatics Association, 20*(3), 470–476. doi: 10.1136/2012-001241

## CHAPTER NINE

# Developing Metrics That Support Projects and Programs

*Andrew Missel and Patricia L. Thomas*

## Chapter Objectives

1. Identify methods that support projects and their management.
2. Identify the importance of organizational culture and evidence-based practice improvement for successful project planning and management.
3. Discuss tools to assess organizational readiness in relation to evidence-based projects and management.
4. Apply tools that capture project milestones.
5. Ascribe a meaning to available data in designing meaningful metrics that result in project sustainment.

## Key Terms

| | |
|---|---|
| Evidence | Metrics |

## Roles

| | | |
|---|---|---|
| Champion | Project manager | Team member |
| Leader | | |

## Professional Values

| | | |
|---|---|---|
| Accountability | Communication | Evidence-based |

## Core Competencies

| | | |
|---|---|---|
| Analysis | Coordination | Representing |
| Assessment | Design | |

# Introduction

At its core, the act of "measurement" is fundamentally about communicating change. The more structured and clear the communication, the more likely the change is to be accepted, supported, sustained, and replicated (Datsenko & Schenk, 2013). Communication can take many forms, ranging from articles with a large national impact that are disseminated through academic, peer-reviewed journal publications to local demonstrations within single inpatient units using dashboards, posted charts, and/or graphs. Regardless of the scale and audience, in today's U.S. healthcare system, one of the most important stories to tell is that of performance optimization and, more broadly, that of quality improvement. These initiatives represent central strategies for improving the value proposition of an often fragmented and inefficient care delivery system (Radnor, Holweg, & Waring, 2012; Waring & Bishop, 2010).

Predicated on three Institute of Medicine reports—*To Err Is Human: Building a Safer Health System* (1999), *Crossing the Quality Chasm: A New Health System for the 21st Century* (2001), and *Health Professions Education: A Bridge to Quality* (2003)—several national imperatives were established. One of the most widely accepted has been the Institute for Healthcare Improvement's (IHI, 2015a) strategy and model created as a framework to discipline improvement work and foster replication of initiatives directed toward patient safety and quality improvement. Based on elements from these activities, a three-step process to guide improvement work has been established: (1) Identify problems or opportunities for improvement; (2) select appropriate measures of these areas; and (3) obtain a baseline assessment of current practices, then remeasure to assess the effects of improvement efforts on measured performance as foundational managing projects within health delivery. The discussion here focuses on the second of these steps—that is, *how to select the right measures for a project or program* and the influence of organizational decision making, culture, and evidence-based practices.

While many examples of healthcare quality improvement frameworks exist in the literature, one of the simplest and most popular is known as the Triple Aim, developed by the Institute for Healthcare Improvement (IHI, 2015b) and illustrated in **Figure 9-1**. This framework suggests that to build lasting and meaningful change, new initiatives must be developed to communicate three sides of the same story:

- The patient experience of care (including quality and satisfaction)
- The health of populations
- The cost of health care

Figure 9-1   The Institute for Healthcare Improvement's Triple Aim.

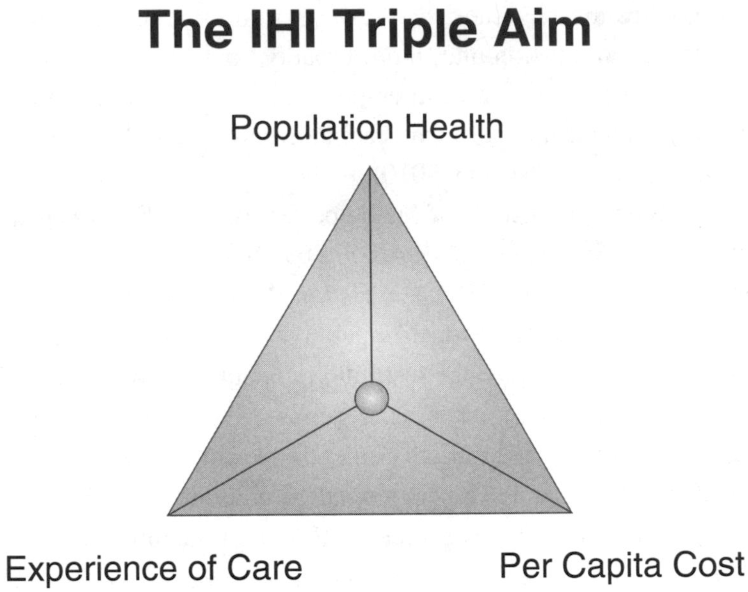

# The IHI Triple Aim

## Population Health

Experience of Care                    Per Capita Cost

*Source:* The IHI Triple Aim framework was developed by the Institute for Healthcare Improvement in Cambridge, Massachusetts (www.ihi.org).

To be successful, the story of a performance optimization project or program, told through the lens of data, must include chapters from all three perspectives. The goal here is to provide simple, actionable instructions on how to weave together that story using data.

## Organizational Culture and Project Management

While the discipline of project management framed by data is critical to project or program success, the culture within an organization or unit cannot be ignored. In recent years, both the "soft" and "hard" sides of leadership and project management have been recognized as key factors, in large part because projects or programs have failed due to their neglect (Radnor et al., 2012; Sheppy, Zuliani, & McIntosh, 2012). Malloch and Porter-O'Grady (2010), Mazurek-Melnyk and Fineout-Overholt (2015), and Nelson, Batalden, and Godfrey (2007) address organizational culture and change leadership as foundational to implementation of evidence-based practices and quality improvement, emphasizing the need to honestly assess the environment to leverage strengths (and champions), and to prepare for resistance or compliance proactively.

Common barriers to successful implementation of projects or their replication include lack of leader champions, insufficient human and fiscal resources, and unrealistic expectations regarding the time necessary for design and achieving desired outcomes. Schein (2004) describes organizational culture and leadership as two sides of the same coin, with both having a significant influence within organizations, particularly when instituting change. Inclusive of the spoken and unspoken values, norms, and espoused beliefs, awareness of the culture is essential to success, but is all too often overlooked at the beginning of a program or project. Setting project goals and developing a charter for the work team that outlines expectations, timelines, and lines of accountability and authority structure expectations is an initial step. What is often missed is the discussion and planning directed toward perceptions, change leadership strategies, and methods to address the team activities that will be undertaken if the agreed-upon changes start to backslide toward the previous state. Each of these entails a distinct strategy for management and requires acknowledgment of the power that culture has in influencing them (Shirley, 2011).

Lam and Robertson (2012) were curious about the ways organizational culture was linked to the success or failure of improvement projects without empiric support for this attribution. They developed and administered a survey to 1027 healthcare employees to investigate perceptions of organizations' culture and willingness to participate in continuous improvement projects. Experience and participation in previous improvement projects, tenure, and organizational demonstration of support for change had a statistically significant influence on individuals' willingness to participate in improvement projects. The use of a disciplined project management structures versus ad hoc project management did not have a significant influence. These researchers' results highlighted how an organization's support for and success in implementing change greatly influenced willingness to participate in improvement projects, which in turn became a part of the organizational culture.

The link to organizational readiness and assessment of this readiness, including data availability, administrative support, and outcome analysts' support, provide organizational information with which to determine how poised a team is to accept change. The rationale for a change readiness assessment or evaluation of the culture provides important information to leaders that can be applied to reduce or eliminate impacts on staffing and caregivers who will be affected by a project (Brown & Hough-Falk, 2014).

## Use of Evidence-Based Practice: An Intertwined Element

*Evidence-based practice* and *evidence-based medicine* are established "buzzwords" that get affirmative nods from many practitioners across disciplinary lines. Despite this affirmation, many disciplines have been slow to adopt evidence-based practices and often identify solutions to problems or new changes to implement without benefit of the **evidence**. For discussions related to selection of **metrics**, project development, and the ensuing evaluation, alignment to evidence in the design of the program or project aims, and in the development of activities or interventions, is essential (Malloch & Porter-O'Grady, 2010; Nelson et al., 2007). Without clarity derived from definitions and reputable evidence found in the literature, in tandem with selection of interventions based in levels of evidence considered acceptable given the scope of the change (or project), replication is difficult, and credibility of outcomes may be questioned (Hall & Roussel, 2014; Mazurek-Melnyk & Fineout-Overholt, 2015). While outside the focus of this chapter, understanding of the model that an organization has selected to evaluate evidence and the framework it uses to implement evidence are important considerations for the project manager to explore during the pre-design work.

Levels of evidence have been established and are generally accepted across the United States. These levels are often depicted as a pyramid. Evidence at the lowest and widest point of the pyramid includes animal research; higher levels of the pyramid are then populated by case studies or reports, case-control studies, cohort studies, randomized controlled trials, systematic reviews, and meta-analysis (at the top of the pyramid) (Hall & Roussel, 2014). Evidence is also often described based on its strength, with expert opinion, experience, theory, and qualitative studies having the least strength; again moving up through a pyramid structure, higher levels consist of non-experimental studies, research studies or randomized controlled studies, and evidence studies as categories at the top of the pyramid. Inherent in this evaluation of strength are components of consistency, quantity, and quality of the evidence (Mazurek-Melnyk & Fineout-Overholt, 2015). It is incumbent upon the project manager and members of the team to consider levels and strength of evidence by using appropriate structures and processes within the organization as projects are designed and progress. Depending on the project or program undertaken, the evidence base that underpins the work may determine the metrics and measures of success.

## Selecting the Right Variables to Tell Your Story

Selecting variables to establish measures of progress and success can be daunting. Members of the project team often come from different disciplines, are prepared through different educational programs, and have different job or role expectations—all of which combine to bring diversity and create a wide space for misunderstandings. For the project manager, one important role is to simplify the process and bring a sense of confidence and inclusion to those completing the work. To that end, using metaphors that infuse common meaning and understanding among team members offers a space for shared learning and understanding. When discussing metrics, measures, and variables, a helpful metaphor for groups who will implement change is that of "telling a story through data." What follows is an example of how "telling a story" can guide variable selection and bring clarity around complex topics.

Take a look at any home library. Most likely, the shelves are a cornucopia of different genres of books. The subjects could range from science fiction and biographies to poetry and romance. Each book tells a unique story from a unique perspective, with a unique cast of characters. This is also the case in health care: There are many unique stories to be told, each with its own unique storytelling style and supporting cast of characters. These stories can be told through the lens of data and measurement. Think of each chart, graph, and dashboard as a chapter of the story being told. Each measure or variable is a different character, with a specific role and perspective. The Agency for Healthcare Research and Quality (AHRQ, 2014) defines three general story genres, each with its own matching style and measurement purpose: (1) quality improvement, (2) accountability, and (3) research.

## Quality Improvement

Measures of clinical quality improvement can be used to illustrate practices within or across an organization, and also could apply to smaller groups such as units or service lines. These measures cover many aspects of patient care such as health outcomes, patient safety, care coordination, and adherence to clinical guidelines. One of the simplest examples of a health outcome measure is the 30-day mortality rate. Another example is the percentage of patients 65 years and older with a body mass index (BMI) greater than or equal to 23. The resulting value is reflective of the quality of clinical service being delivered to the patient population.

## Accountability

Measures of accountability support the needs of audiences other than those who directly provide care, such as payers, regulators, accrediting organizations, and patients. The results may be used, for example, to compare provider groups, select providers based on performance, or establish a case for providing financial rewards (AHRQ, 2014). One example of a measure of accountability is the percentage of advanced practice registered nurses (such as certified nurse-midwives) in a given service line (OB/GYN, for example). This metric is a measure of nursing quality and professional development within a specified service line, and could be used by the department to make decisions about nurses' pay scales.

## Research

Measures for use in clinical research differ from quality improvement and accountability measures by their intended use. The primary use of measures in research is to generate new knowledge that is generalizable (AHRQ, 2014).

These insights may be valuable in setting health policy, evaluating programs, or assessing the effectiveness of a clinical practice or guideline, though the last typically requires larger sample sizes and more detailed data collection. Very often, the collection of data for use in clinical research will require the engagement of an institutional review board (IRB) to enforce ethical or patient safety guidelines.

## Fundamental Types of Measures

### Process Measures

Measures of clinical process describe "activities carried out by health care workers to deliver services" (AHRQ, 2014). Such measures reflect specific and observable aspects of clinical practice. A prominent example comes from emergency cardiac care. For patients presenting to the emergency department with ST-segment elevation myocardial infarction (STEMI), door-to-balloon time measures a process that starts with the patient's arrival and ends with an intervention performed in the cardiac catheterization laboratory. This process measure describes the total time necessary to complete a series of processes associated with treating a patient with STEMI, which are carried out by multiple care team members. A key feature of process measures is that they can be easily and clearly defined. As a result, when properly defined, process measures are generally not adjusted based on case mix or risk level.

Information about completed processes emerges from two sources. First, the process can be directly observed. Staff with a stopwatch can time how long it takes to complete a specific task or shadow clinicians to determine whether a specific task is completed. This practice is referred to as upstream measurement— the measurement is taken *as the action is being completed.* One example is the observational audit of staff to ensure that proper hand washing procedure is followed.

Alternatively, downstream measurements may be generated from information on processes that *have already been completed.* With this type of measurement, data are often extracted from administrative sources such as patient charts or the electronic medical record. Door-to-balloon time for STEMI patients is an example of downstream measurement because the measure is reported as a the sum of the time it takes to complete multiple processes, which is typically extracted from the medical record after the patients comprising the sample population have been discharged. Another example is the examination of patient charts to see if fall prevention education was delivered. The chart review takes place after the process of delivering fall prevention education should have been completed.

Downstream measures have two important limitations that cannot be overlooked. First, they typically indicate only whether a process was completed—a binary ("yes/no") indicator, lacking any qualifiers. They do not clearly indicate *how* the process was completed. Expanding on the example of fall prevention education, using a downstream measure for this process would not reveal any information about how much time was taken to speak to the patient and gives no indication whether the patient fully comprehended the information provided—two pieces of information that could have been captured if the process had been directly observed. Second, downstream measurements introduce recall bias by relying on staff to record information after the task has been completed, sometimes several hours later. For these reasons, upstream measurement is the preferred option where available, but should be balanced against the greater demands placed on the cost of gathering this data (such as staff time and expense).

## Outcomes Measures

Although representing different viewpoints, both measures of process and measures of outcomes must be included to tell the complete story of any project or program. Outcome measures are the cornerstone of quality improvement. For many projects and programs, improving patient outcomes is the final goal. Outcomes capture a variety of health states like mortality, physiologic measures (blood pressure, laboratory test results), and patient-reported health status (functional status and symptoms) (AHRQ, 2014). These variables represent final goals of clinical interventions and processes—that is, improved health status for patients or populations.

Process measures and outcomes measures are intrinsically linked. One of the most common mistakes made in measurement strategy is the conflation of the two. For example, evaluating a care management training program on medication reconciliation in primary care practices considers two separate issues: (1) the process measures derived from the training process and (2) the outcomes or results of this training on medication reconciliation as the outcome. It is not uncommon, however, for these distinct measures to be described as one entity. In developing a project or program, calling out the distinctions between process and outcomes is essential so that appropriate measurements and clarity around accountability and results can be determined.

## *Qualitative Measures*

While quantitative measurement is most commonly used based on its specificity and the ease of data gathering and analysis, qualitative measurement offers a different perspective. Measures that tell the story of a stakeholder's opinion about a process are called qualitative measures because they convey deeper meaning regarding the quality, or how *well*, a given process was fulfilled. A plethora of qualitative measures can be found on the Hospital Consumer Assessment of Healthcare Providers and Systems (HCAHPS survey; also known as the CAHPS Hospital Survey). HCAHPS provides national, standardized, publicly reported survey results of patient perceptions of care received during a hospitalization (Centers for Medicare and Medicaid Services [CMS], 2014). This 27-question survey about a patient's recent hospital stay is administered to a random, monthly sample of all eligible discharges. One example qualitative measure from this survey tool is the percentage of patients who report that their nurses "always" communicated well during their stay (H-COMP-1-A-P). This measure is considered to be qualitative because it reflects a person's opinion about nurse communication—what is considered to be "good" or "effective" communication varies from person to person. Similar surveys exist for home and hospice care (HHCAPS).

## Selecting the Right Data

When possible, measure sets are best focused on the patient or individual, commonly referred to as "patient-centered" measures. When read together, such measures show how a patient or population of patients progresses through a given process or disease state. This simplifies understanding and provides a platform for replication.

## Matching Populations

When selecting sets of variables, care should be taken to use the same time frame and the same target population across the entire set. Mismatches of this type are, unfortunately, common. Using **Table 9-1** as a reference, there would be little insight to be gained by reporting the average length of stay for a population of patients discharged between the months of January and June at the same time as 30-day all-cause mortality rate for patients discharged between the months of July and December. By definition, these are two different populations with two different stories to tell. The resulting noise makes interpreting any trend, change, or intervention outcome difficult, and it may even be impossible to discern any differences. In addition to reporting time frames, other mismatches

**Table 9-1** Sample Inpatient Heart Failure Measure Set

| Variable Description | Data Source | Measure Type |
|---|---|---|
| Heart failure and shock with major complications (MS-DRG 291) | CMS (ICD-10-CM) | Outcome; quantitative |
| Heart failure and shock with complications (MS-DRG 292) | CMS (ICD-10-CM) | Outcome; quantitative |
| Heart failure and shock without complications or major complications (MS-DRG 293) | CMS (ICD-10-CM) | Outcome; quantitative |
| Average length of stay (ALOS) | Administrative clinical data; EMR | Process; quantitative |
| 30-day, all-cause mortality rate | Administrative clinical data; EMR | Outcome; quantitative |
| Patients discharged to ambulatory care or home health care | Administrative clinical data; EMR | Process; quantitative |
| 30-day, all-cause unplanned readmission rate | Administrative clinical data; EMR | Outcome; quantitative |
| Patients who received heart failure education | Administrative clinical data; EMR | Process; quantitative |

can arise in terms of the underlying population (different groups of patients) and processes without connection or causal relationship. Drawing conclusions about the impact a change has when the "noise" is not accounted for can lead to attributions that are distorted or inaccurate.

## Benefits of Using Established Measures

Many of us are tempted to write or establish individual data definitions as a means to highlight the uniqueness of an organization or a patient population. This practice may occur because individuals recognize that currently available data are valued by those engaged in the project or because certain data are readily available. Often, individuals look for ways to stimulate buy-in, particularly when the "charge" or expectation to make meaningful change originates outside the work team that is expected to generate the change. While tempting, this undertaking requires knowledge and analysis not generally found in healthcare organizations and should be avoided if national or specialty-specific data definitions already exist. Over the last decade, significant progress has been made in establishing evidence-based, validated, credible data definitions that promote comparability within a single facility or with other organizations, especially when participating in regional or national quality improvement collaboratives.

## Common Data Sources

Examples of evidence-based, validated measure sets abound.   Organizations such as those listed below, offer comprehensive lists of measures from which to choose.  Many source the data for their publicly reported performance measures from organizational administrative and claims data.  Carefully consider how a measure set matches the specific process, outcome, discipline or population you are investigating.

- CMS
- National Database of Nursing Quality Indicators (NDNQI)
- AHRQ National Quality Measures Clearinghouse
- Organizational administrative and claims data

## *Eliminating Unnecessary Measures*

In the Lean and Project Management Body of Knowledge (PMBOK) method-ologies, any work that adds cost or time, or that expands the scope of the work without adding value, is considered to be wasteful. One specific type of waste that is applicable to measurement strategy is called overprocessing. Overpro-cessing can take many forms, including requesting and processing more infor-mation than is necessary or information that will never be used, or reporting duplicative information (Hadfield et al., 2012). A central tenet of the Lean meth-odology is to measure only that which one intends to impact through a project or program. Eliminating waste from your dashboard—in the form of vestigial or unnecessary variables—will increase the clarity and impact of the story being told. Additionally, and perhaps more importantly, this streamlining will increase the ability to glean new knowledge such as trends from the data, which could otherwise be hidden behind the noise of unnecessary measures. For example, if the goal of a program is to establish a process for complex care coordination in the emergency department (ED), the measurement of ED median arrival-to-discharge time adds no valuable information.

To eliminate waste from an established dashboard of measures, begin by clarifying the reporting and communications needs of involved stakeholders. Look for measures that do not include information being expressly requested. This step is also a centerpiece of change management: If stakeholders are not involved early in the process of making changes, there is a higher risk that dis-ruptions could arise later in the project life cycle.

## Summary

- In this era of health reform where both cost and quality garner equal attention, it is incumbent on members of the healthcare profession to develop skill and confidence in measuring (quantifying) the impact of their work.
- For many healthcare professionals, the prospect of selecting metrics in-stills fear because of these measures' importance in creating a powerful story to share with others about the contributions nurses make with their

work. Recognizing the stature of nurses within the healthcare delivery system, *The Future of Nursing: Leading Change, Advancing Health* (a 2010 report written by the Robert Wood Johnson Foundation and the Institute of Medicine) identified, as a key message, the need to partner fully with members of the healthcare team and improve the information data infrastructure to support decision making and policy making directed to improved health outcomes for the United States. Inherent in this recommendation is the ability to manage projects, establish evidence, and distinguish appropriate metrics and measurement for change outcomes.

- As the U.S. healthcare delivery system is reformed, an essential lever will be measuring meaningful elements of healthcare practice to improve outcomes.
- Building from what has been learned about research and evidence-based practice implementation, the disciplines of project management and quality improvement serve as the guardrails for selection of meaningful metrics.

## Reflection Questions

1. Consider the definitions of process and outcome indicators. Select an area of practice where you believe a project could be developed. What are some of the process metrics you might consider to demonstrate progress or improvements in care? What are some of the outcome measures you would consider?

2. You are having lunch with a colleague who works on a different unit. She has heard about a program that is being developed to serve the patient population you care for. She does not understand how the decisions were made about data that will be analyzed. How would you explain the decision-making process for selecting metrics?

3. Reflect on your current practice. Where would you go to get information about data available in your organization? Data in the electronic medical record? Administrative data? Claims data? Data sets or a data warehouse? Who are the people (or roles and departments) who can help you develop knowledge and understanding of the available data?

# References

Agency for Healthcare Research and Quality (AHRQ) National Quality Measures Clearinghouse. (29 May 2014). Uses of Quality Measures. Accessed 11 Jan. 2015 at http://www.qualitymeasures.ahrq.gov/tutorial/using.aspx.

Brown, B., & Hough-Falk, L. (2014). Embarking on performance improvement. *Healthcare Financial Management, 68*(6), 98–103.

Center for Medicare and Medicaid Services (CMS). (25 September 2014) HCAHPS: Patients' Perspectives of Care Survey. Accessed 17 January 2015 at http://www.cms.gov/Medicare/Quality-Initiatives-Patient-Assessment-Instruments/HospitalQuality-Inits/HospitalHCAHPS.html

Datsenko, Y., & Schenk, J. (2013). Leading clinical projects. *Applied Clinical Trials Online,* 22–28. http://images.alfresco.advanstar.com/alfresco_images/pharma/2014/08/20/c6374106-d388-4605-8d9c-95cee53438fc/article-821735.pdf

Hadfield, D., Holmes, S., Kozlowski, S., Sperl, T, & Tapping, D. (2012). *The new lean healthcare pocket guide: Tools for the elimination of waste in hospitals, clinics, and other healthcare facilities.* Chelsea, MI: MCS Media, Inc.

Hall, H., & Roussel, L. (2014). *Evidence-based practice: An integrative approach to research, administration, and practice.* Burlington, MA: Jones & Bartlett Learning.

Institute for Healthcare Improvement (IHI). (2015a). How to Improve. http://www.ihi.org/resources/Pages/HowtoImprove/default.aspx

Institute for Healthcare Improvement (IHI). (2015b). The IHI Triple Aim Initiative: Better care for individuals, better health for populations, and lower per capita costs. http://www.ihi.org/Engage/Initiatives/TripleAim/Pages/default.aspx

Institute of Medicine (IOM). (1999). *To err is human: Building a safer health system.* Washington, DC: National Academies Press.

Institute of Medicine (IOM), Committee on Quality of Health Care in America. (2001). *Crossing the quality chasm: A new health system for the 21st century.* Washington, DC: National Academy Press.

Institute of Medicine (IOM). (2003). *Health professions education: A bridge to quality.* Washington, DC: National Academies Press.

Lam, M., & Robertson, D. (2012). Culture, tenure, and willingness to participate in continuous improvement projects in healthcare. *Quality Management Journal, 19*(3), 7–15.

Malloch, K., & Porter-O'Grady, T. (2010). *Introduction to evidence-based practice in nursing and health care* (2nd ed.). Sudbury, MA: Jones and Bartlett Learning.

Mazurek-Melnyk, B., & Fineout-Overholt, E. (2015). *Evidence-based practice in nursing and healthcare: A guide to best practice* (3rd ed.). Philadelphia, PA: Wolters Kluwer.

Nelson, E., Batalden, P., & Godfrey, M. (2007). *Quality by design: A clinical microsystems approach.* San Francisco, CA: Jossey-Bass.

Radnor, Z., Holweg, M., & Waring, J. (2012). Lean in healthcare: The unfilled promise? *Social Science & Medicine, 74,* 364–371.

Robert Wood Johnson Foundation & Institute of Medicine. (2010). The future of nursing: Leading change, advancing health. http://www.thefutureofnursing.org/sites/default/files/Future%20of%20Nursing%20Report_0.pdf

Schein, E. (2004). *Organizational culture and leadership* (3rd ed.). San Francisco, CA: Jossey-Bass.

Sheppy, B., Zuliani, J., & McIntosh, B. (2012). Science or art: Risk and project management in healthcare. *British Journal of Healthcare Management, 18*(11), 586–590.

Shirley, D. (2011). *Project management for healthcare.* Boca Raton, FL: CRC Press.

Waring, J., & Bishop, S. (2010). Lean healthcare: Rhetoric, ritual and resistance. *Social Science & Medicine, 71,* 1332–1340.

# Case Exemplar

## ■ CASE STUDY 1

### Bachelor of Science in Nursing Scholarship Program

*Summer Li and Patricia Thomas*

## Background

As part of the national health system, nurse leaders wanted to create a process to work toward the Robert Wood Johnson Foundation and Institute of Medicine's *Future of Nursing* report (2010) recommendation of having 80% of the nursing workforce with a bachelor is science in nursing (BSN). "Every clinical outcome targeted for improvement over the past year in U.S. hospitals has been definitively linked to the degree of nursing educational preparation and training" (RWJF & IOM, 2010). Research shows that a high percentage of BSN preparation among registered nurses (RNs) is associated with better patient outcomes (Rambur, Palumbo, McIntosh, & Mongeon, 2003). Feedback from chief nursing officers (CNOs) and staff has identified differences in tuition support and long periods between starting a BSN program and completing it as obstacles to achieving the IOM's goal. Several of the barriers relate to the difficulty of paying for college courses "up front" given other financial and family responsibilities that take priority.

The CNOs and executives of a large national health system committed to increasing the percentage of BSN staff in the workforce across the system. The CNOs established several strategies, including BSN preferred hiring, support of BSN education through local university on-site BSN completion programs, and support from the health system's foundations for ongoing education. Another prong of the strategy included the development of a BSN scholarship program with two schools of nursing—one that was owned by the health system, and one that was a strategic partner.

The purpose of the BSN scholarship programs was to provide funding resources through scholarships that would enable registered nurses holding a diploma or associate degree obtained via online programs to acquire BSN degrees. Scholarship recipients would "pay back" the organization for the upfront money by working full time for the organization for three years (or six years if working part time). There was recognition that building a stronger nursing workforce would result in better quality outcomes, patient safety, RN retention, patient satisfaction, and associate engagement.

The BSN scholarship program was unique in that it functioned as a loan program. Scholarship recipients need to commit to completing the program within two years and fulfill the service requirements at their hospital after graduation before the loan could be forgiven. This arrangement added complexity to the project in several areas.

## Risk Management, Stakeholder Management, and Communication Management

Given the nature of the loan program, the legal and tax implications needed to be clearly identified and managed. It was critical to involve the right stakeholders up front to design the program and ensure that it met all legal requirements. In addition, ongoing management of the scholarship recipients required collaboration between nursing education and human resources (HR) personnel. Consequently, a multidisciplinary team was developed, including stakeholders from legal, finance, accounting, nursing leadership, and human resources from both the system's centralized office and local hospitals. The team members worked together to identify risks and solutions/processes to avoid or minimize risks.

In the governance structure of the project, all key stakeholders were selected and assigned to the steering committee, advisory group, and work group with different responsibilities. One of the key stakeholders in the process was the hospital-based BSN scholarship liaison. This person was responsible for ensuring all the loan documents were properly signed and executed, connecting scholarship recipients with other parties, and tracking the status of those recipients and their fulfillment of the service requirements after graduation. Ongoing meetings were set up to review the process and loan documents, and to provide onboarding education to new liaisons. All needed information was posted on the health system's intranet to provide easy access to those interested in the BSN program. A frequently asked questions (FAQs) document was also provided to address common concerns and questions from scholarship recipients.

# Process and Continuous Improvement

A small team was convened to identify each step in the process to ensure all the parties involved were well connected. The program was centrally managed at the system office, including the following functions:

- Providing loan documents templates and related education to hospitals
- Paying tuition to the nursing school
- Charging the tuition back to hospitals with scholarship recipients

Hospitals were responsible for managing the scholarship recipients' personnel files and tracking the fulfillment of their service requirements. All the required documentation was put into a documentation checklist based on different scenarios and shared with hospital contacts for further action.

With any ongoing project, it is important to keep continuous improvement in mind. In the three years since the program's initiation, the program has gone through the plan–do–check–act (PDCA) cycle. After the first year of implementation, an annual evaluation was conducted to collect feedback and lessons learned. Based on that information, an annual planning process was put into place to provide hospitals with all the important days (i.e., deadlines) and tasks for the entire year in one document. It significantly improved the team members' efficiency and helped hospitals establish their timelines and processes for selecting scholarship recipients. In addition, all the loan documents are subject to legal review on an annual basis to ensure compliance with legal requirements in each state and to minimize the legal risks.

# Lessons Learned

One of the challenges in this project was that not all hospitals were on the same HR system. Lack of standardization among the hospital HR systems made it impossible to centrally manage the scholarship recipients' status and their fulfillment of the service requirements. Eventually, hospitals took responsibility for managing those pieces. In fact, striving for standardization of HR and other supporting systems will significantly improve efficiency.

Another challenge was communication, which is not unique to this project. Changes in the hospital BSN scholarship liaison personnel have occurred on a regular basis. It has been found to be critical to ensure the smooth transition and effective onboarding education. The old saying really is true: "Communicate seven times and seven ways."

## Metrics and Measures for the Project

Many people had different ideas of meaningful metrics and measures for the project. The team chose two outcome metrics—number of nurses enrolled and number of nurses graduated—which were reconciled on an annual basis. Several metrics were used to communicate progress throughout the academic year, and were shared with both the schools of nursing and the CNOs: enrollment numbers, courses completed, dates on which payments were made (and charges back to the hospital), and number of scholarship recipients selected by each hospital each semester. While many process metrics could have been selected to establish progress, these were the indicators selected by the CNOs, the liaisons, academic partners, billing and finance staff, and senior executives of the hospitals.

## Reflection Questions

1. The RWJF & IOM's *Future of Nursing* report identifies a recommendation for BSN-prepared nurses. Which role can you play to ensure this recommendation is met?
2. Consider your current work setting and the culture for lifelong learning. How can you influence stakeholders to support the advancement of nursing?
3. How can continuous improvement advance nursing and interprofessional teamwork?

## References

Rambur, B., Palumbo, M.V., McIntosh, B., & Mongeon, J. (2003). A statewide analysis of RNs' intention to leave their position. *Nursing Outlook 51*(4), 182–188.

Robert Wood Johnson Foundation & Institute of Medicine. (2010). The future of nursing: Leading change, advancing health. http://www.thefutureofnursing.org/sites/default/files/Future%20of%20Nursing%20Report_0.pdf

## CHAPTER TEN

# Measuring the Value of Projects Within Organizations and Healthcare Systems

*Patricia L. Thomas and Michael Bleich*

## Chapter Objectives

1. Define value in relation to clinical project planning and management.
2. Describe strategies for aligning value with projects.
3. Identify the principles of project evaluation.
4. Discuss methods to disseminate project value.

## Key Terms

| | | |
|---|---|---|
| Evaluation | Information | Quality improvement |
| Evidence | management | |

## Roles

| | | |
|---|---|---|
| Communicator | Leader | Project manager |
| Data analyst | Planner | Stakeholder |

## Professional Values

| | | |
|---|---|---|
| Autonomy | Integrity | Social justice |

## Core Competencies

| | | |
|---|---|---|
| Assessment | Evaluation | Synthesis |
| Critical thinking | Leadership | Systems thinking |
| Design | Management | |

# Introduction

When an organization undertakes a project, it is typically aligned to an aspect of the mission and vision statement or the current strategic plan. Resources, usually constrained, are invested and used, which means that these same resources are being shifted from other parts of the organization and other projects. This simple frame belies the essence of this chapter—that value must be defined, attained, and demonstrable by measurement to ensure that the resources did, in fact, advance the organization's mission and vision. Likewise, the investment of resources in any project should produce value for the organization's stakeholders—notably patients, families, staff, physicians, clinical service staff, employees of the organization, payers, regulators, and the board of directors.

Measuring value is difficult both conceptually and practically. First, measurement requires the use of information, usually drawn from databases but often collected specifically for a project, based on the anticipated outcomes of the project. The information collected must be informative, meaning that a pre-designed plan for its use has been determined. If it informs, then it must also be relevant to the project and sensitive so that it measures real differences in the project's anticipated impact. Further, information must be unbiased and comprehensive to capture the scope and magnitude of the project. When these criteria are met, the integrity of the project's impact is established as real and cogent.

Measuring the impact of a project also requires timely information. Attention must be paid to how and where information is stored and maintained so that impact can be measured throughout the project's duration. In project management, information must be performance-based, targeted to the goals and objectives of the project, collected in a uniform manner, obtainable with relative ease, and—importantly—cost-effective (Hall & Roussel, 2014).

The next challenge is how to capture value. Value is different from cost, in that it serves to meet a perceived need of a stakeholder. Value is expressed by first identifying the stakeholder's interest. In the case of a project that influences organizational efficiencies, this interest may be measured in time saved, simplification of a complex task, replacement of a way of working that is distasteful with one that is the opposite, supplanting of one method by another, and the like. Dimensions of cost-effectiveness, job autonomy, and other factors may also contribute to perceived value (Malloch & Porter-O'Grady, 2010).

The project manager must be clear about the stakeholders' needs and wants to establish the appropriate baseline for comparison of outcomes. Similarly, if the project impacts patient care, then the patient's perceptions must be considered. Will the project facilitate access to care? Or will it provide for symptom management, influence quality of life, diminish pain or discomfort, or reduce the advancement of disease to a higher stage of chronicity? The project leader must be clear about the aim of the project and establish this from a value perspective

(Harris, Roussel, & Thomas, 2014). As stated earlier, measuring value is complex and requires considerable forethought and design.

As this discussion makes apparent, the project manager will play multiple roles in measuring the value of projects within organizational settings. Indeed, measuring the value of impact in any project must be considered even before the project is initiated. The project manager must understand the genesis of the project, especially when a senior leader delegates a project or when a project is aligned to an element of the organization's strategic plan. Leaders may view the project as an opportunity to demonstrate their professional acumen and skills in change leadership. As such, project managers need to consider the cultural context of the work. Which organizational dynamics led to the project? What are the strategic and operational impacts desired from the project? Who are the affected stakeholders? What will be lost in the creation of change, and what will be gained as a result of the project? The role of leadership is evident as the project team ventures into the unknown. The role of manager is executed by guiding the project through a defined process. But additional roles germane to this chapter are also relevant: The project manager must be strategic and must function as a planner, a communicator, a data analyst, and even a database administrator. Value, then, based on stakeholder expectations, may be expressed in terms of time saved, cost, convenience/access, and simplicity of use.

## Aligning Metrics with Project Aims

Projects vary in terms of the magnitude and scope of the change, the stakeholders involved, and the degree of linearity or complexity associated with the approach taken to manage the project. **Table 10-1** provides a useful framework for examining a project's level of complexity (Berger, 2005). Strategies for project implementation and means by which value may be created warrant special attention. As complexity increases, the number of individuals and groups with their own expectations about and definitions of value will inevitably grow as well.

An example of a simple project might be the introduction of a product that is available at the point of care to encourage hand hygiene. The aim of the project has a defined location (bedside), a defined targeted audience (bedside caregivers), and a targeted aim (nosocomial infection reduction or prevention).

**Table 10-1**  Project Characteristics as a Precursor to Metric Selection

| Simple Project | Mid-Range Project | Complex Project |
|---|---|---|
| Stakeholders are limited to a select few, often with readily aligned values and needs. | Stakeholders are modest in number and cross boundaries within an organizational setting where values and needs are similar. | Stakeholders are large in number or are of varying disciplines with often disparate values and needs. |
| The project is primarily linear with clearly defined outcomes targeted at individuals and groups. | The project is both linear and nonlinear in that the outcomes extend to influence behaviors that are less defined and that focus on the group level of attainment. | The project is primarily nonlinear with a less-defined structure, and the outcomes cannot be clearly defined and are aimed at social change. |
| The project manager retains the ability to oversee and control each aspect of project activities. | The project manager works with a team to oversee and provide general direction while the project unfolds and morphs to meet unanticipated needs. | The project manager does not exist in one individual, but rather extends to intersecting groups, all of which share a common aim; multiple strategies emerge to shape the direction of the project. |
| Metrics are simple to retrieve from existing data and can be readily observed or collected; feedback loops are easy to define and often stem from a single source. | Metrics are retrieved from multiple data sources and may require development beyond what is available, with feedback loops required from multiple sources. | Metrics are retrieved from large databases and public opinion and must capture the multiple interests within divergent populations and stakeholders. |
| Metrics focus on project completion and simple outcomes. | Metrics focus on organizational impact and more complex outcomes, beyond project completion to project impact. | Metrics focus on social change with complex social outcomes. |
| The value to measure is tied to a few defined concepts within a narrow range. | The value to measure is tied to multiple concepts within a broad organizational range. | The value to measure is tied to social concepts that cross organizational boundaries. |

*Source:* From Berger, S. (2005). *The power of clinical and financial metrics: Achieving success in your hospital.* Chicago: Health Administration Press, pp. 150

As simple as this project might seem, the project leader must consider what to measure and answer certain questions. For example, should hand-washing compliance using the product be measured? Should changes in nosocomial infection rates be measured? Is the impact of the product measurable in real time or retrospectively? Is there an existing database from which to draw information? Does a database need to be created? Will one sample be used for outcomes, or will the entire population be included in the analysis? When is the best time to collect the data to represent the results with integrity and to reduce risk? Who will collect the data, and how will data collection be coordinated? As these questions and potentially others suggest, the complexities of measuring value are endless.

## Teams, Engaging Experts, and Oversight

While the project manager is responsible for the design, development, and oversight of the work undertaken, it is not uncommon for a project manager to work with a team (either a team created for the specific project to be implemented or a team that previously existed but has been tasked with the current project). To that end, project management requires awareness of team dynamics, the ability to facilitate diverse groups or teams, and the objectivity to identify when experts or outside consultants are needed to achieve the aim or goal of the project. Inherent in these role responsibilities is the need to maintain a clear line of communication with the person who delegated the project. Navigating lines of authority and accountability is a task undertaken at the onset of the project, which must be clearly articulated, documented, and communicated to all who will participate in the work (commonly through a charter or specific aims document).

## Principles of Project Evaluation Methods

Project **evaluation** is the effort made to measure the impact of project-based change. The value proposition to be measured is derived from the stakeholders themselves, who are often highly diverse. One stakeholder (a shareholder) may have a singular interest in profit. Another stakeholder (a patient) may have an interest in access, cost, and quality. Regulators may seek adherence to a defined set of standards. Many projects evolve from **quality improvement** initiatives, where metrics are similar to project management metrics. In fact, the principles of developing metrics for quality improvement serve as a substantive guide for project evaluation (Finkler, Jones, & Kovner, 2013; Malloch & Porter-O'Grady, 2010).

To adequately meet the needs of the stakeholders, the project manager must fulfill the responsibility of measuring the impact of project objectives or aims. These objectives should readily be aligned with the organization's mission and purpose if the level of change is targeted within an institutional setting. Some projects extend to multiple settings, however; they are therefore more complex to evaluate than when a single value proposition is being assessed. Insurance companies may have a desire to provide different health education, for instance, than what is desired in the provider–patient relationship. These differences in stakeholders' interests must be accounted for in complex changes.

Some researchers perceive project evaluation methods as being closely aligned with the field of program evaluation. Program evaluation is a diligent investigation of a program's characteristics and merits to provide information about its effectiveness in optimizing the outcomes, efficiency, and quality of health care. Evaluations can analyze a program's structure, activities, and organization and examine its political and social environment. Foundationally, evaluation appraises the achievement of a project's goals and objectives and the extent of its impact and costs (Lewis, 2011).

Project and program evaluation differ from other types of research in that their major task is to identify a program's merits. Developing value metrics in an organizational context, then, can relate to measuring program objectives and activities, program outcomes, and program impact.

Methods used to capture data include both quantitative and qualitative strategies. Quantitative methods include approaches that measure impact through mechanisms such as data retrieval from existing administrative and national databases, economic cost-effectiveness determinations, surveys measuring perceptions, and targeted research instruments that measure patient, family, and societal outcomes that align with the project objectives and aims. Examples of quantitative data include selecting metrics from the following sources:

- Clinical/epidemiologic databases, disease registries, or epidemiologic surveys
- Administrative claims data at the organization or state level
- Sociodemographic data available in census reports or state-level vital statistics records
- Patient satisfaction data from proprietary databases at the institutional level
- National Data on Nursing Quality Indicators (NDNQI) data at the institutional level
- Marketing data that specify lifestyle and other useful population practices

Similarly, qualitative data provide a rich context for evaluating project impact. These data are available through the following sources:

- Focus groups with project-oriented aims
- Appreciative inquiry/storytelling methods aligned with stakeholder groups
- Internet and social networking approaches to capture context

## Information Dissemination: Roles and Responsibilities for Communication

The project manager has the ultimate responsibility for ensuring that the impact of project implementation is reflected in useful ways to stakeholder groups. As early data are collected, the dissemination of information is critical to the stabilization of the project. Those engaged in the change need and want feedback on how the project is progressing. While the full impact of change may be unknown in the early stages of data collection, it does provide motivation toward meeting project aims and objectives.

Face-to-face communication is helpful, but when it comes to data presentation, it is insufficient. Consequently, the project manager displays data using charts, survey tools, graphs, and other means to fully reflect the impact of the project during its implementation and at the conclusion of the intervention, and continues to monitor post-intervention effectiveness and restabilization. Today, electronic support of data presentation and analysis underscores the need to be transparent in all facets of program accountability.

Rarely do projects turn out exactly as planned. If the right metrics are selected—namely, those that are sensitive to the project aims and objectives—and if the data are reliably collected and displayed, then variations from the plan will likely occur. This does not mean the project has failed, but rather presents an opportunity for the project leader and stakeholder groups to "torture the data" (to use John Ruskin's eloquent turn of phrase), such that meaning emerges from the data. In other words, data themselves do not signify success or failure of a project. Only analysis of their collective meaning with an eye toward improvement can settle the question of a project's success. All too often, however, project managers feel the obligation to measure that which appears to denote success rather than to capture what is successful—or not—about a project.

The presentation of feedback through quantitative and qualitative data offers the opportunity for the project leader to anticipate risk, integrate findings with lived reality, communicate a sense of purpose to the stakeholders, and design plans for improving the project past its due date and weaving it into the fabric of the work of the organization.

Especially in the case of projects that lead to system change, the use of statistical process control charts helps to determine the impact of the change and resets the new and improved standard, such that variation can be identified as either being created by the system change itself (known as common-cause variation) or representing a major aberrancy that rests outside of the system change (special-cause variation) (Deming, 1986; Keller, 2011). These techniques, which are used in quality improvement, are critical to help determine whether a changed system is performing in a desirable manner and quickly draw attention to special causes that are not related to the change itself. Although outside of the scope of this chapter, statistical process-control tools should be part of project managers' toolkit to aid in decision making and direction setting (Keller, 2011).

Lastly, it is important to portray the effects of change to stakeholder groups. A final report, a summary email, a closure event to mark achievements, and the publication of run charts with notes attached to denote accomplishments are all mechanisms that can be employed to tell the story of the value that the project brought to the organization, its stakeholders, and others who evaluate the organization, such as external regulators, public constituency groups, and the like. Today, nurse leaders are not present often enough in the boardroom to discuss change, but a well-educated project leader, with the right tools for communication and data presentation, should make an appearance in this venue to advance patient care and to inform others of the contributions of nursing and other healthcare professionals.

## Tools of the Trade

In project management, inexpensive statistical process-control software is readily available. Some basic analytic procedures can be performed with an Excel spreadsheet, for example. When such tools are used, the process changes that have occurred can be monitored for common-cause and special-cause variation, as described previously. The control chart that emanates from statistical process control powerfully documents change and variability (Keller, 2011).

Similarly, graphic presentation of data is useful, particularly when the data can be modeled in a dashboard style of presentation. A dashboard presentation compares and contrasts metrics into a single document, such that patient outcomes, staff performance, economic data, and risk data, for example, can be studied as a set, aiding decision making by highlighting that one variable (e.g., cost savings) is not working against other variables (e.g., patient satisfaction). This is another important tool for decision making and evaluation (Carroll, Flucke, & Barton, 2013).

## Professional Considerations and Expectations

Healthcare reform, change, pay for performance, and public reporting have become the norm in the healthcare realm in the last decade. Given these trends, complexity has become a part of the care delivery landscape, and clinicians and leaders continue to search for guideposts and consistency in a rapidly changing world. Advance practice nurses have assumed the responsibility for leading interprofessional teams through disciplined and consistent activities to achieve organizational goals.

Inherent in the ability to lead others through change are a deep understanding of physical and social sciences, critical thinking skills, and the ability to design, implement, monitor, and evaluate programs or projects (American Association of Colleges of Nursing [AACN], 2006, 2011; Quality and Safety Education for Nurses [QSEN], 2012). The Robert Wood Johnson Foundation and Institute of Medicine's *Future of Nursing* report (2010) has established an interdisciplinary expectation and set of core competencies for patient-centered care built on best **evidence**, continuous (and consistent) quality improvement, and the use of data analytics to guide intervention. Master's- and doctorate-prepared nurses are positioned through education and experience to demonstrate the awareness and openness necessary to leverage critical thinking, team building, and requisite synthesis of complex situations to establish foundational and replicable strategies for decision making. The capabilities necessary to accomplish these goals will include the ability to influence others through formal and informal communication, relationships, and reputation. Teaching, mentoring, and coaching other members of the healthcare team will be requisite skills—skills present in nurses' current practice and historically relied upon by others.

One of the greatest challenges facing any healthcare discipline and members of an interprofessional team will be the ability to incorporate the principles and discipline of quality and process improvement before looking for solutions. Balancing quality of care, financial pressures, and efficiency will be essential while preserving clear alignment to one's ethical obligations. Historically, organizations have focused their change actions on quality, cost, or efficiency as a singular interest, often at the expense of the other areas. The work facing organizations and project leaders requires equal and disciplined attention to each of these arenas simultaneously (AACN, 2006, 2011; QSEN, 2012).

## Summary

- Value is obtained by knowing the specific stakeholder wants and needs related to the project. These can vary widely, but often include access to service, cost-effective delivery of service, and satisfaction with the project's outcomes.

- Metrics encompass the art and science of measuring value. Metrics must be informative, relevant, unbiased and comprehensive, action-oriented, performance-targeted, and cost-effective. Projects vary in complexity, and the metrics employed in those projects will vary accordingly. Metrics can include both quantitative and qualitative data, which are complementary concepts: Whereas the former provides information about specific points of achievement, the latter provides context.
- Project leaders are accountable for a fair and honest representation of the project and should be prepared to reveal progress toward the project's aims, as well as unanticipated outcomes, both positive and negative.
- The utilization of decision-science tools, such as statistical process-control charts and dashboard maps, to represent work and adapt projects is fundamental to project management; these instruments are the expected tools of the trade.

## Reflection Questions

1. What is the importance of defining a clear end-point vision prior to implementing a project? Which role should stakeholders play in articulating this vision?
2. Which role does standards setting play in selecting metrics? Does Donabedian's structure → process → outcome model have any relevance in choosing metrics?
3. How do the research principles of data validity and reliability tie into data collection in project management? Should data that do not have confirmed validity and reliability play any role in evaluation?
4. How does one determine the cost of data collection and management compared to its relative value in project evaluation?

## Learning Activities

1. Take an existing project and determine whether clear outcomes for the project were stated early on in the project. Examine who the stakeholders were and who they should have been to establish these outcomes.

Did a data collection plan exist that would measure the impact of the project?

2. Develop measurable and obtainable metrics for a project. For each metric, identify an operational definition that focuses on what the metric measures and how it ties to the project. Develop a sampling plan for data collection, including deciding whether the data will be collected in real time or on a retrospective basis. Determine who will collect and display the data and whether the data will come from an existing database or must be collected as new data.

3. Prepare a plan for using the data at various phases during and after the project. Anticipate how the data will affect decision making and provide feedback to stakeholders.

# References

American Association of Colleges of Nursing (AACN) (2006). The essentials of doctoral education for advanced nursing practice. http://www.aacn.nche.edu/publications/position/DNPEssentials.pdf

American Association of Colleges of Nursing (AACN). (2011). The essentials of master's education in nursing. http://www.aacn.nche.edu/education-resources/MastersEssentials11.pdf

Berger, S. (2005). *The power of clinical and financial metrics: Achieving success in your hospital.* Chicago, IL: Health Administration Press.

Carroll, C., Flucke, N., & Barton, A. (2013). The use of dashboards to monitor quality of care. *Clinical Nurse Specialist*, 61–62. http://www.cns-journal.com, doi: 10.1097/NUR.0b013e31828191b5

Deming, W. E. (1986). *Out of the crisis.* Cambridge, MA: MIT Press.

Finkler, S., Jones, C., & Kovner, C. (2013). *Financial management for nurse managers and executives* (4th ed.). St. Louis, MO: Elsevier Saunders.

Hall, H., & Roussel, L. (2014). *Evidence-based practice: An integrative approach to research, administration, and practice.* Burlington, MA: Jones & Bartlett Learning.

Harris, J., Roussel, L., & Thomas, P. (2014). *Initiating and sustaining the clinical nurse leader role: A practical guide* (2nd ed.). Burlington, MA: Jones & Bartlett Learning.

Institute of Medicine. (2010). Future of nursing: Leading change, advancing health. http://www.iom.edu/Reports/2010/The-Future-of-Nursing-Leading-Change-Advancing-Health.aspx

Keller, P. (2011). *Statistical process control demystified.* New York, NY: McGraw-Hill.

Lewis, J. (2011). *Project planning, scheduling, and control* (5th ed.). New York, NY: McGraw-Hill.

Malloch, K., & Porter-O'Grady, T. (2010). *Introduction to evidence-based practice in nursing and health care* (2nd ed.). Sudbury, MA: Jones and Bartlett Learning.

Quality and Safety Education for Nurses (QSEN). (2012). QSEN competencies for advanced practice nurses. http://www.aacn.nche.edu/faculty/qsen/competencies.pdf

## Suggested Readings

Henriques, S. (2010). The project management simplicity method. http://www.scribd.com/doc/27897513/Project-Management-Simplicity#scribd

Management Centre. (2015). Organizational development: Appreciative inquiry. http://www.managementcentre.co.uk/downloads/AppreciativeInquiry.pdf

# Case Exemplar

## ■ CASE STUDY 1

### Healthcare and Community Agency Partnerships

A project manager has been appointed based on a community desire to be more heart-healthy. The hospital responded favorably to this community request, which emanated from several organizations including the YMCA, the statewide affiliate of the American Heart Association, and civic leaders whose concern was a healthy workforce. A cardiovascular nurse leader was selected by the hospital's chief executive officer (CEO) to lead the hospital's efforts to make a huge impact on cardiovascular health. The project aims included assuring that exercise was available to all age groups on a year-round basis, having one or more citizens trained in cardiopulmonary resuscitation (CPR) reside on every city block, and placing a defibrillator device in all public buildings with an occupancy of 75 or more people. Fortunately, these project aims were all measurable, which is not always the case.

The nurse leader charged with leading this project had a number of complex design challenges to think through, so beginning with a willing spirit and having strong personal values that supported the project was a good thing! Using Table 10-1 as a reference, the nurse determined that components of the project could be subdivided and that they crossed over all project levels from simple to complex. The nurse leader recognized that the project had dimensions that addressed social justice and included an altruistic component. Evidence about cardiovascular disease supported the project and could be used for ideas about measuring the project's impact. Evidence that did not already exist also needed to be gathered. The following questions needed to be answered:

- How many establishments exist that accommodate 75 or more people? How many have automatic external defibrillators?
- How many city blocks exist, and where do the city limits end? Does the charter really mean city blocks, or should suburbs be included? What are the ramifications if they are not included? What is the anticipated risk of limiting the project to the city?

- How does one define exercise? What are socially acceptable norms relating to exercise given weather conditions and public safety issues? How will the communities of interest value and accept the risks associated with exercise or the lack thereof?

Only when these and similar questions were answered could an effective metric design and **information management** plan emerge.

Systems thinking was needed by the nurse leader to understand the interrelated components of the project and to recognize which parts of the project had linear, systematic, and predictable components to them versus which aspects of the project targeted larger social and policy issues. In a brainstorming session around metrics, the following suggestions emerged:

- Collect data on satisfaction with CPR training.
- Count the number of individuals who exercise on a regular basis.
- Look at the number of heart-related procedures that are performed at the local hospital and see if they decrease.
- Look at claims databases to check for cardiac risk factors.
- Mandate that vending machines have their food choices altered to include healthy alternatives and count the changes.
- Count the number of people who attend a health fair and have their blood pressure taken.
- Restrict public smoking because of its link to heart disease, and monitor heart disease occurrences.
- Count the number of new exercise programs that are held in public places, including long-term care facilities.

## Reflection Questions

1. If one was planning to use this list of suggestions, how useful would it be?
2. Which data are tied to simple, mid-range, and complex social change?
3. How accessible is the information suggested? Is it performance targeted? Is it new or existing data? How does it tie to the project objectives?
4. How do the metrics suggested integrate with the project? What would you change?

# ■ CASE STUDY 2

## A Value-Based Project Crossing Disciplines

*James L. Harris*

Jane, a graduate student in an executive administration program at a local university, was assigned a clinical project to be completed in two semesters. Jane had often pondered how she could engage others to improve care for adults in an acute psychiatric unit where she was employed on a part-time basis. More specifically, patients who were admitted to the psychiatric unit and later experienced the need for intravenous fluids (IV), oxygen therapy, and IV antibiotics were transferred to medical or surgical units. Frequently, prescribed psychiatric medications were discontinued upon transfer, so return of the patients' psychiatric symptoms quickly ensued. Staff from the psychiatric unit were reassigned to the medical unit to provide care when behavioral interventions were required. Not only did this result in additional costs in overtime for the psychiatric division, but interventions also followed to resolve behavior problems exhibited by the transferred patient, often due to medication discontinuation.

Jane was sure she had a great opportunity to develop a business case for resolving the need to transfer patients to medical or surgical units. Her first task was to discuss the project with the nurse manager, unit director, psychiatric and medical chiefs and residents, nursing staff, quality director, team members from other divisions, educators, engineering, and patients. Each of the conversations focused on quality, safety, and value directed at patient centered care. This data informed the needs assessment that followed.

Through a rigorous process of discussions, cost analysis, and focus groups with various individuals and patients, a business plan was developed and approved by the chief executive officer of the facility. The following months included a series of planning sessions, retooling of psychiatric nurses' duties and skills to handle medical issues, and construction. Based on the data, four to six medical/psychiatric beds were needed on a daily basis to avoid transfer of patients for IV and oxygen therapy.

Within six months of the plan's approval, four medical/psychiatric beds were opened. A myriad of positive outcomes followed, including close dialogue among medical and surgical residents and attending and psychiatric staff daily, the employment of a nurse practitioner, staff engagement from all disciplines, no transfers to medical units, greater satisfaction among patients and families, cost avoidance, and reduction in injury of medical and surgical nurses when transferred patients exhibited hostile behaviors.

What started as a project vision resulted in a quality, safe, and value-based intervention that led to interprofessional dialogue, interventions, satisfaction, and patient-centered care delivery. The four-bed success later resulted in conversion to four additional medical/psychiatric beds and additional services offered. The value extended far beyond cost avoidance to a sustainable and highly functional unit.

## Reflection Questions

1. What roles do communication and stakeholder buy-in play in the success of a project?
2. How can a project planner ensure that value is measurable in any project? Identify the key measurement components.

## CHAPTER ELEVEN

# Disseminating Results of Meaningful Projects and Their Management

*Catherine Dearman*

## *Chapter Objectives*

1. Identify methods for dissemination and effective management of projects for diverse audiences.
2. Discuss techniques and drawbacks when disseminating project plans, implementation, and data outcomes.
3. Discuss methods to disseminate project value using an executive summary, abstract, editorial, and professional development portfolios.

## *Key Terms*

Dissemination                 Presentations

Posters                       Publication

## *Roles*

Audience                      Speaker

Presenter                     Team member

## *Professional Values*

Professionalism

## *Core Competencies*

Communication        Leadership              Professionalism

## Introduction

No one does the work entailed in a project or innovation just to complete it; sharing the outcomes and lessons learned with others is a natural result of all the work and effort. In many situations, **dissemination** of the work is essential to sustainability of the project or innovation. Without dissemination, others within the organization and outside it will not be sufficiently aware of the project, which may impact the program's use and overall outcomes. Some projects naturally lend themselves to replicability within the system by the same team or similar teams, as well as in other systems. Replicating a project can yield distinct positive results and serve to integrate the findings into the system, thereby improving sustainability. Sustainability and replicability are inextricably linked to projects and the teams that produce them.

Dissemination of the results of projects and creative work is aimed at promoting the exchange of information and extension of the work. It is essential to sustain the innovation and to spread the outcomes into various outlets. Dissemination of designs, processes, and outcomes allows others to truly understand the project and to determine how a similar project might work in their system. Replication of the project itself is not necessarily the goal; rather, dissemination provides a sample or a plan as to how any innovation can be completed.

Dissemination can take many forms and to some extent depends on the venue in which the project took place. Nurse educators and those in the academic setting typically focus on the **publication** of articles in journals or the production of papers or **posters** for verbal presentation. Clinicians and nurse executives, in contrast, may seek to share their works at a more local or practice-based level. Many facilities working toward Magnet status must not only demonstrate that they have participated in quality improvement projects, but also show that the processes and results of those projects have been disseminated and sustained throughout the system. Larger healthcare systems use projects and other creative and innovative works to advance team members on a career ladder. Dissemination is an integral part of all of those processes.

The true impact of a practice project or innovation is not always limited to one or more healthcare systems. Some innovations are best shared through social media, on blogs, and even in "lay" literature such as women's or men's magazines.

This chapter addresses the dissemination of processes and outcomes through multiple venues and provides real-world information on preparing and delivering data to various groups and in a myriad of settings. The focus is on structuring the dissemination and methods of ascertaining submission requirements as well as on designing the actual dissemination itself. Dissemination is positively impacted when each person knows and deliberately uses skills to enhance delivery of the data. Use of a systems approach and appreciative inquiry methods will provide an opportunity to capitalize on the skills and talents of the various team members who collectively produced and are disseminating the work.

## Professional Presentations

Most formal and many informal **presentations** involve the use of audio, audiovisual, or supportive technology, such as Microsoft's PowerPoint program, flip charts, story boards, video, and posters. Presenters must always be aware that equipment may fail, be incompatible with the venue, be cumbersome, or be lost in transit; it is therefore critical to have a backup. The literature is replete with models or strategies to structure a presentation. Acronyms provide an easy method to remember the components the speaker needs to address in preparing a presentation. APPLE: audience, presentation, purpose, language, and evidence, provides a ready structure that is amenable to any presentation whether one will address a group of students, peers, or an international gathering

### *Audience*

Consideration of the audience is critical to an effective presentation. The audience aspect of the APPLE model can comprise the intended audience or the actual one. The intended audience is the group you are intending to reach, while the actual audience is the individuals who are exposed to the presentation. In any given venue, one may prepare a presentation for a group of like-minded individuals—but the attendees may not share the same view and, therefore, may respond in unexpected ways to the presentation. The presenter needs to be prepared to address the audience (intended or actual) effectively and manage the interaction in order to have a successful presentation.

### *Presentation*

The presentation itself can be oral or written and may or may not include visual aids. Most presentations are planned, but some may take the form of spontaneous, off-the-cuff sharing of data. For example, a faculty member may be walking across campus when he or she is approached by a student or group of students who pose a question. The resulting dialogue could be termed a presentation of data, though little about it would be considered formal.

Personal preference and presentation style as well as the venue itself will guide whether the presentation is formal or informal. In some cases, a full paper is presented along with a verbal presentation. The paper is then included in a "proceedings" document for the conference. Proceedings documents count as publications, doubling the benefit to the presenter. A research conference venue would naturally require statistical methods and data outcomes to be presented in a rather formal style. A conference designed to showcase teaching strategies or unit-specific interventions would highlight various teaching strategies and engender dialogue.

## Purpose

The purpose of the presentation has two possible aspects: explicit and implicit. The explicit purpose is the stated reason for the presentation; the implicit purpose is what the presenter actually hopes to accomplish. For example, one may verbally express a primary purpose of a presentation as being to share the processes and outcomes of the project or innovation. The implicit purpose may be to further the presenter's career through sharing their scholarly work. The presenter's implicit purpose will, to some extent, shape the presentation and can make or break the outcome when combined with consideration of the audience and the presentation style.

## Language

The language component refers to the level of diction and formality; voice and tense; objectivity versus self-reference; and scientific/professional versus lay terminology or street language. The evidence or the information being conveyed can impact the language used in the presentation. It may be supported by data, facts, opinions, direct observations, references to the work of others, and hearsay, among other forms.

The presenter is responsible for tailoring the language to the audience and the venue. Failure to do so can negatively impact the entirety of the presentation.

### *Engagement*

Engaging the audience can entail maintaining eye contact, positive facial expression, and asking questions and eliciting responses, either verbal or non-verbal. Other methods of engaging the audience include assuring that objectives match content, that the abstract or description provided to a potential audience is congruent with the actual presentation, and maintaining a less formal style.

Remembering APPLE will facilitate the speaker being able to structure an effective presentation. Other considerations for podium presentations include honoring time constraints imposed by the conference to facilitate smooth operation. Extending over time impacts both audiences and other speakers.

Presentations may also occur as a group event or a panel discussion. In those cases, the time frame is for the entire group, not for each individual speaker. Participating as a part of a group or a panel typically means a far more restricted environment resulting in less opportunity to tailor the presentation to the individual speaker.

Visual and/or auditory aids are typically included along with the oral components of the presentation. Many speakers embed short videos or short computer interactions that make their point effectively and efficiently. If including these adjunctive methods, the speaker must be aware of the software and hardware interfaces available at the conference. Embedding a critical auditory or visual aid that is not effective in the venue can have a significant negative impact on the presentation.

## Role of Appreciative Inquiry in Presentations

Appreciative inquiry (AI) is the co-evolutionary search for the best in people, their organizations, and the relevant world around them. Appreciative inquiry gives life to a living system; presentations using AI provide an opportunity to share the hidden aspects of a system or a project that are not obvious to the audience. AI includes the art and practice of asking questions that strengthen a system's capacity to apprehend, anticipate, and heighten the positive potential from a project or innovation (Cooperrider & Whitney, 2010).

Traditionally, a project is not communicated until it is completed, and an innovation is not considered complete until outcomes are communicated. In AI, communication of outcomes occurs throughout the entire process of innovation, thereby creating transparency and an evidence-based culture (Marchionni & Richer, 2007). The approach to be used to communicate outcomes requires forethought, flexibility, willingness to capitalize on the differing presentation strengths of team members, and the ability to view the innovation process entirely.

The personal style of the presenter is critical to an effective presentation. The component of personal style addresses the unique strengths and characteristics that blend well with different people and situations at different times. Identifying and capitalizing on one's strengths and matching them to the characteristics of the intended audience increases the opportunity to make a truly successful presentation. When presenting early findings, matching one's personal style with the intended audience is especially critical. Early findings are more tenuous and can be ambiguous. Even skilled presenters can be challenged if the audience is not receptive to the data. Presentation of information about an innovation is considered successful if the information is remembered favorably and implemented or applied to new situations.

Personal style includes personal appearance, ease of interacting in different settings, vocal qualities (including volume, tone, pitch, and intonation), and personal power. Habitual and deliberate use of gestures, ease of making eye contact, ability to listen, ability to communicate interest and enthusiasm about the topic, and willingness to accept criticism can either add to or detract from a presentation. Being aware of one's personal style is essential to making effective presentations (Rutledge, Bajaj, & Mucciolo, 2007).

Ensuring the sustainability of an innovation requires understanding the various factors that influence its dissemination. Appreciative inquiry provides the context for disseminating results that directly contribute to sustaining innovations within systems by making the implicit connections more explicit. In other words, sustainability rests on presentations making essential hidden connections more obvious for all to see. The result is transparency for the team, the system, and the audience (Havens, Wood, & Leeman, 2006).

# Publications

Publications in academic circles are more valuable than other types of data sharing, such as posters, books, and book chapters. In this context, the word "publication" typically refers to an in-print paper that appears in a peer-reviewed journal. "Peer-reviewed" indicates a level of quality review that exceeds that performed in non-peer-reviewed or any other type of publication. Other terms indicating a peer review are "refereed" (as in "contested and emerging victorious") and "juried" (as in "from a jury of one's peers"). Academicians, especially those in competitive systems, consider only peer-reviewed publications when making tenure and promotion decisions. Although online publications are becoming more mainstream, print journals remain at the top of the academic pecking order.

Tappen (2011) provided the following advice for would-be authors seeking publication of their work in peer-reviewed journals: Endure criticism, maintain staying power, and tolerate revision. Seldom is one's paper accepted without revision. Other advice regarding peer-reviewed publications includes choosing the journal wisely (i.e., read the articles in the journal, look at the purpose and types of articles typically published, and tailor the submission to those elements). Additionally, authors should read and follow the journal's requirements; compile the literature review properly; organize the paper appropriately with headings and other elements; proofread, proofread, proofread; format the manuscript correctly and double-check it; be willing and able to change the manuscript based on reviewers' comments; and refuse to concede defeat.

Books and book chapters are valuable learning and sharing tools, especially for those professionals early in their career or for health systems. Books and book chapters contain more of the surrounding details than can be shared in a poster or podium presentation and, therefore, are extremely useful for teaching others and for developing a strong writing style.

Posters are useful as mechanisms to share a lot of information quickly. A poster typically consists of a problem statement, findings, data elements, and outcomes. The poster presenter must consider how to provide these elements in a visually pleasing manner that is easy to read and understand (**Figure 11-1**). Poster sessions are frequently held during a conference at lunch or during breaks

Figure 11-1    Sample poster format. Landscape format is desired for display.

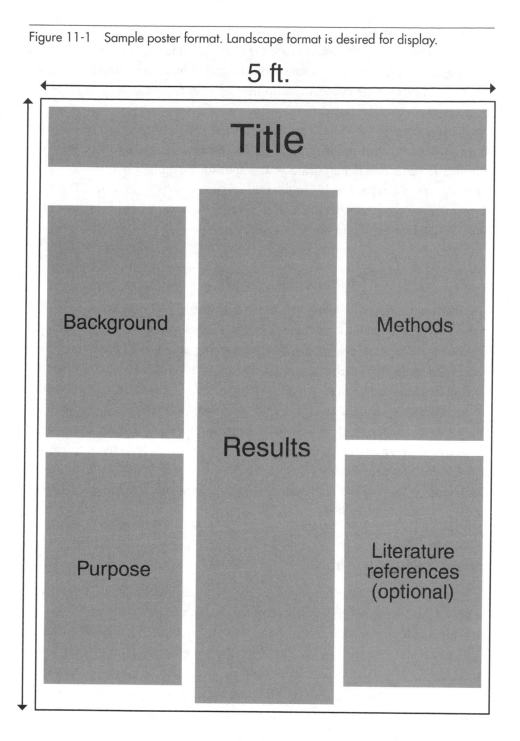

to allow larger exposure of presentations than can be accommodated with paper presentations. Poster presentations are far more informal and occur many times in a one-to-one fashion as interested audience members approach and read about the study. Handouts are especially helpful for poster presenters because they allow viewers to take the presentation with them.

Professional publications, presentations, books/chapters, and posters all share some commonalities in terms of preparation, such as tailoring the submission to the audience, being aware of the sponsor's requirements and assuring that they are followed, and being tolerant of suggestions to improve. The final element is perhaps the most difficult to accept, especially when someone considers himself or herself to be the "expert" on the topic.

## Other Types of Publications

Lay literature can be a valuable teaching tool for the general public. Academicians, however, would not presume to count a submission to a women's magazine or a newspaper as evidence of being deserving of tenure or promotion. That being said, publications that reach a wider population can be quite impactful, especially when the goal is to share "need-to-know" health information or to propose lifestyle changes. Many practitioners will find publication in lay journals to be as challenging as publication in peer-reviewed journals. Not only is the venue different, but the purpose and the manner in which the information is produced are vastly different. The same advice applies when submitting a manuscript to this type of publication: Know the reputation and readership; follow directions; proofread; and take criticism well.

## Social and Informal Presentations

Social networking, such as via blogs, wikis, email, and face-to-face sharing, can be very valuable for disseminating a project. Today, many people can be reached through social media rather than through more traditional methods. In social networking, the message is more personal, and more reflective of opinion based in evidence rather than limited to the evidence itself. In all social networking, presenters must be keenly aware of the audience, group dynamics, and spread of information.

Written reports can be very valuable means of sharing information within a system, especially if one seeks to sustain the project or innovation. This type of publication requires the author to make a more businesslike and more streamlined presentation. A business case must be made and arguments formulated to achieve sustainability. Written reports are frequently shared with internal and external audiences such as external regulators. Above all, the author of such a report should avoid verbosity and adhere to the system's guidelines.

Press releases for television, radio, and newspaper can be another valuable tool for sharing information in a more informal fashion to a more selective audience. However, if you are being interviewed in these venues rather than writing the script yourself, be aware that you may be misquoted or "bumped" if a bigger story occurs. To avoid being misquoted, make an attempt to get review privileges prior to publication; you may encounter resistance from the media outlet because timing is critical, but such a review can save you from heartache.

## Pitfalls in Dissemination

It is critical to be aware of two major pitfalls that can occur with any sharing of information: redundant publication and self-plagiarism. Sometimes an innovation is innovative only for one's own system and is widely accepted outside that system. Becoming an expert on the information contained in the broader literature will prevent this error.

Self-plagiarism occurs when the researcher shares the same information with more than one publication or in more than one presentation. Typically when one is invited to present or publish, the conference or the journal becomes the owner of the information shared. Subsequent publication or presentation of the data, even if you are the researcher who discovered the findings, is problematic. Focused presentations and publications that present one or very limited amount of information can prevent this faux pas and can result in multiple publications and presentations, all different, from a single study, project, or innovation.

Because dissemination requires an ongoing exchange of information between and among project staff, specific planning for dissemination and audiences must be addressed at the inception of project development. Several factors and conditions affecting dissemination, adoption of a project's outcome, and sustainability of the project must be included in all presentations: the advantages that the innovation has brought to the organization; the compatibility of the innovation with the organization; the complexity of the innovation; the ability to track and observe the elements of the innovation; the inherent risks to the project; the expected reversibility and ability to revise each individual element and the project as a whole; and the leadership and support of the organization. All of these elements are based on effective communication within the organization and an assessment of the agency's readiness to change.

## Summary

- Dissemination of innovative projects is a natural progression of any endeavor.
- Project dissemination offers audiences new knowledge and opens up an exchange of information.
- A number of forums are available for dissemination of information, including journal publications, book chapters, and poster and podium presentations.
- Multiple presentation methods and models are available; however, the APPLE model is widely used by individuals to prepare presentations.
- Presentations using appreciative inquiry provide opportunities to share aspects of a system or project that may not be obvious to the audience.
- Careful consideration should be given to where one publishes and presents findings, who maintains the copyright, and which pitfalls of dissemination may be encountered.

## Reflection Questions

1. How does one prepare for a publication or presentation opportunity?
2. Which personal characteristics can impact a presentation or poster?
3. What are three common issues with dissemination of findings from projects?

# References

Cooperrider, D., & Whitney, D. (2010). A positive revolution in change: Appreciative inquiry. http://appreciativeinquiry.case.edu/intro/whatisai.cfm

Havens, D. S., Wood, S. O., & Leeman, J. (2006). Improving nursing practice and patient care: Building capacity with appreciative inquiry. *Journal of Nursing Administration, 36*(10), 463–470.

Marchionni, C., & Richer, M. C. (2007). Using appreciative inquiry to promote evidence-based practice in nursing: The glass is more than half full. *Nursing Leadership, 20*(3), 86–97.

Rutledge, P. A., Bajaj, G., & Mucciolo, T. (2007). Special edition: Using Microsoft Office Powerpoint © 2007, Indianapolis, IN: QUE.

Tappen, R. M. (2011). *Advanced nursing research: From theory to practice.* Sudbury, MA: Jones and Bartlett Learning.

# Case Exemplar

## ■ CASE STUDY 1

### Presentations Supplemented with PowerPoint
### Tips and Examples

*Catherine Dearman*

PowerPoint is an instructional design tool for presentation that is commonly used, especially in business and academic settings. Because PowerPoint presentations are extensions of the traditional presentation, the typical rules for presenting evidence apply. The information that follows provides novice presenters with essential information related to PowerPoint presentations.

A PowerPoint presentation is an adjunct to the verbal presentation, and as such needs to supplement—not replace—the presenter's oral discussion. Most instructional design specialists indicate that there should a maximum of one slide for each minute scheduled for the presentation. This basic setup includes the introductory slide, the reference slide, and the "Questions?" slide.

The basic rule of thumb for slide makeup is to include 7 lines of text with 7 words on each line (at most), for a total of 49 words per slide. At its best, the PowerPoint slide serves as a guide, prompting the presenter to mention salient points. The slides are not expected to contain every word that a presenter needs to say.

Inclusion of pictures on PowerPoint slides can be great, especially if they link to the topic at hand. For example, if the presentation is addressing community work groups building a playground, including before, during, and after pictures would give a complete image to the audience and would replace words.

Most audiences typically prefer lighter backgrounds with darker text. Colors should complement, not detract from, the presentation.

Slide layouts sometimes intrude on the words the presenter wanted to show on the slides. Previewing the slides carefully prior to finalizing the layout will facilitate clarity and attractiveness.

Slide transitions, animation, and sound are all effective attention-getting devices. Use them cautiously, however. Not every slide needs a transition for each word. Flashing words are distracting to some viewers.

Prior to a presentation where visual aids (including PowerPoint slides) are used, the presenter is well advised to assess the environment of the presentation. Go into the room and look around. How many chairs are there? How large is the space? Is it square or rectangular? Are there impediments to full view of the screen, such as poles and projectors? Following this inspection, load the presentation onto the computer and project it. Go to the back of the room and see if the slides are clear or if adjustments in font or other elements are needed. Sometimes a color scheme for a slide looks great on a personal computer but does not communicate as well in a large group.

If the presentation is a result of funding, the funding agency typically prefers to be mentioned in some way. Some funders actually publish the statement they want used with every publication and/or presentation. Be sure to include these statements if they exist.

# INDEX

**Note:** Page numbers followed by *b*, *f*, and *t* indicate material in boxes, figures, and tables respectively.